THE
DIVINE CODE
OF LIFE

THE DIVINE CODE OF LIFE

Awaken Your Genes

&

Discover Hidden Talents

Dr. Kazuo Murakami

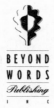

BEYOND
WORDS
Publishing
I N C

Beyond Words Publishing, Inc.
20827 N.W. Cornell Road, Suite 500
Hillsboro, Oregon 97124-9808
503-531-8700
503-531-8773 fax

English translation by Cathy Hirano

Editor: Julie Steigerwaldt
Managing editor: Henry Covey
Proofreader: Marvin Moore
Cover and interior design: Carol Sibley
Composition: William H. Brunson Typography Services

Printed in the United States of America

ISBN-13: 978-1-58270-144-8

The corporate mission of Beyond Words Publishing, Inc.:
   Inspire to Integrity

Contents

PREFACE

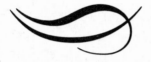

To my readers:

In October 2004, I was invited to participate with nine other scientists and visionaries in the "Dialogue between Buddhism and the Sciences," a biennial meeting hosted by His Holiness the Dalai Lama at his residence in Dharamsala, India. The Dalai Lama had read about my research on how laughter affects genes and has taken a keen interest in it. The actor Richard Gere, who was a guest at the meeting, evinced great interest in my presentation. This book covers almost everything we discussed at that meeting.

Research in the life sciences is advancing at an astonishing pace, exceeding even the expectations of those who work in this field. The human genome was completely decoded just a couple years ago. We now have the necessary means and skills to read the blueprint of the human body. Although at first we believed that the cracking of the genetic code would solve the mystery of life, it has become increasingly clear that life is not so simple. The more we study even a single cell, the more we understand its immense complexity. I have been involved in life science research for over forty years, the latter half of which has been devoted to genetic research. The goal of this book is to convey the inspiration, surprise, and wonder I have derived from both the content and process of that research and to share with you how you can apply some of those insights to how you live your own life.

There are two points in particular that I wish to share with you. The first is the remarkable discovery that our genes are not fixed but change in response to various factors. How many people in the world blame their shortcomings, such as a lack of aptitude at sports, on their parents? It is true that heredity influences individual characteristics and abilities. But although these traits are genetically transmitted, our genes also come equipped with an on/off switch that can change their function. Regular exercise, for example, switches on good genes that result in improved muscle tone and health and, at the same time, switches off harmful genes.

The environment can also trigger this on/off mechanism. From what I've observed in research and in my own experience, exposure to a different environment seems to stimulate good genes and unlock a person's potential. Even more amazing, however, is the fact that the on/off mechanism can be triggered by mental attitude. Research now shows that our way of thinking can activate our genes. A recent experiment I led, which I will describe in detail later, found that laughter significantly reduced blood-sugar levels in diabetics after meals. We subsequently identified specific genes that are activated by laughter, proving for the first time that positive emotion can flip the genetic switch. Learning how to activate positive genes and deactivate negative genes could open up infinite possibilities for expanding human potential.

The second point presented in this book is a scientist's perspective on what makes possible all the wonder around us. The enzyme/hormone system and the related genes that govern hypertension have been the focus of my life's work. Yet despite almost a century of extensive research by many capable scientists, much remains unknown about even this single subject.

The mechanism of life is an amazing mystery. People talk about "living" as if it were a simple matter, but not a single human being could survive by conscious effort alone. Regulated by the automatic functioning of hormones and the automatic nervous system, all our vital functions, including respiration and blood circulation, work full time to keep us alive without any special effort or intervention on our part. It is our genes that control these vital systems, and to do so, they work in perfect harmony. When one begins to function, another responds by stopping or by working even harder, fine-tuning and regulating the system as a whole.

It seems highly inconceivable that such superb order could occur by mere coincidence. Something greater must be behind the harmony of our world. Many use the word *God* to describe this concept; as a scientist I have chosen to call it "Something Great." Although it is invisible and not easily perceived with our other senses, working as I do in the field of life sciences, I am strongly aware of its existence. Cracking the genetic code is a truly marvelous feat; yet even more marvelous is the fact that this code was imprinted on our genes in the first place. We know that we did not write it, yet it cannot have been written randomly. The genetic code, which is equivalent in volume to thousands of books, is contained within and mysteriously yet undoubtedly controls the infinitesimal space known as the cell.

It is human nature to seek to know the unknown and to strive to understand the incomprehensible. "What's new?" is the scientist's constant refrain, demonstrating that the destiny of science is to evolve. As long as our fundamental curiosity does not change, science will continue to progress. New developments and discoveries in the life sciences, in particular, have immediate effects, leading to new technology, to improved breeding techniques in livestock farming, or to the creation of new medicines. As a result, however, science and technology can be easily perverted to satisfy avarice and personal ambition. Accordingly, if we do not find some way to control baser human desires, science will forever remain a double-edged sword.

The central issue in the debate concerning human clones is not technology but rather human greed. How far should we go? Is it appropriate to create a physical copy of yourself merely because you want to? Science and technology make it possible, but it is people who decide whether or not to do it, and more often than not that decision is based on selfish interests. We should not be so arrogant. Rather, we should remember that life, including our own, is a gift from "Something Great" and not the product of human invention or greed.

We need self-restraint, the ability to refrain from doing something unnatural even if it is technically possible. But self-restraint is insufficient if it is based solely on ethics. Self-restraint is born from the knowledge that we live not by our own strength or devices but rather by the grace of a myriad other lives that support our own. By living with gratitude and appreciation for this gift we can activate our dormant genes and open the door to a new and wonderful way of life.

As the founder of the Institute for the Study of the Mind-Gene Relationship, I am pursuing research to prove my hypothesis that happiness, joy, inspiration, thankfulness, and prayer can activate beneficial genes. The result of the experiment on laughter mentioned earlier represents our first discovery. Our research, as it progresses, could offer an explanation for the truths taught by the Buddha and the Christ described in terms of the genetic on/off mechanism.

If I had dared to say that positive feelings can activate genes twenty years ago, I would have been harshly criticized for being unscientific, but the number of scientists who share my perspective on the power of the mind is increasing. In fact, scientists all around the world are conducting experiments to understand how psychological factors influence the physical. We need to end the misconception that the mind is unrelated to physical well-being. Until that time, it will be difficult to eradicate diseases with conventional scientific methods alone. As scientists and as part of an international community, we need to devote more effort and resources to studying the mind. In the world we live in today we encounter many problems without easy solutions. It is crucial to have science and spirituality working together, complementing each other, if we wish to find the answers. I hope that this book will be of service in this regard.

In my quest for understanding, I have been fortunate to encounter many wonderful people. I am particularly indebted to Dr. Reona Ezaki, Nobel Prize laureate and former president of Tsukuba University; and Dr. Hisateru Mitsuda, professor emeritus of Kyoto University and my lifelong mentor, for their guidance over many years. I take this opportunity to express my heartfelt gratitude.

I would like to thank His Holiness the Dalai Lama for his endorsement of my research. I would also like to express my sincere appreciation to Richard Cohn and Cynthia Black of Beyond Words Publishing, Inc., and translator Cathy Hirano for their assistance in publishing this book. The Japanese version has sold over 200,000 copies, and I am eagerly looking forward to the response of English-language readers to the ideas I will share.

Kazuo Murakami

INTRODUCTION

Recent advances in the rapidly evolving field of genetics have attracted worldwide attention. The development of genetically modified vegetables has generated concern about whether or not such foods are safe to eat, while the birth of a cloned sheep and other mammals has sparked controversy concerning the possibility of identical human clones.

We have a preconceived notion of what "genes" are, but in fact we know very little about them. Until a few decades ago, the term *heredity* was almost synonymous with fate or destiny. The characteristics passed down from one generation to the next were seen as immutable. Statements like, "It's heredity; there's nothing you can do about it," expressed the futility of fighting against the inevitable. People assumed, for example, that a child born to musically gifted parents would be blessed with musical ability while a child born to diabetic parents would have a much higher risk of developing the disease. Likewise, it was believed that children of overweight parents would become obese and children whose parents had cancer would probably die of it too. Such things still tend to be regarded as fate.

Of course, ability can be developed with great effort, and the effects of unfavorable genes can be mitigated through strict control, but it has been difficult to argue with someone who insists that a particular trait, regardless of whether it is good or bad, is "hereditary." Recent genetic research, however, has resulted in an extraordinary discovery. Because genetics is the study of life itself, every new discovery is extraordinary, but this one is directly related to you. Experiments by myself and other scientists have shown that the environment and other external factors can actually change the way our genes work. To be more precise, we now know that dormant genes can be activated.

When speaking of the environment or external stimuli, people tend to think in material terms, but I include the psychological level as well. The effects of psychological stimuli or trauma on our genes—in other words, the connection between our genes and our minds—have been gaining attention and will continue to do so in the future.

Numerous phenomena in the world around us point to the existence of this connection. A severe shock, for example, can cause a person's hair to turn white in a single day. Conversely, a terminal cancer patient informed that he has only a few months to live may live six months, a year, or even many years longer. Someone who has never smoked a cigarette in his life may get lung cancer, whereas another who has smoked a hundred cigarettes a day may be extremely healthy. Although eating too much salt should cause hypertension, a person who loves salty food may have normal blood pressure.

We also know that people under extreme conditions can exhibit superhuman strength or that falling in love can transform a poor student into a hard worker who suddenly excels at his studies. These things happen all the time, and people have found many different reasons to explain them. In fact, all of these phenomena are directly related to how our genes work, and the outcome can change depending on the attitude of the individual.

We see this potential all around us, although we may not recognize it for what it is—the power of the mind at work. We know, for example, that the nature of a cancer can change depending on whether the patient thinks, "I'm going to get better," and focuses all her energy on this belief, or whether the patient thinks, "I'm going to die," and gives up entirely. Similarly, someone with severe hypertension who is convinced that he has low blood pressure will actually have fewer symptoms.

At this point in time, the concept that these phenomena are deeply related to our genes is still in the realm of hypothesis, but there is much circumstantial evidence to support it. With continued research, it's my belief that the effects of our psychological state on our genes will be clarified in the near future.

There is no need, however, to just wait idly for that day to arrive. If knowledge can contribute to a better life, we should take advantage of it now. It is with this aim in mind that I wrote this book—to share with you useful and fascinating information that I have learned from my work with genes.

The Wonder of the Genetic Code

In addition to causing cell division and transmitting characteristics from parent to child, genes work ceaselessly at a much more immediate level. We could not speak, for example, without the functioning of our genes, which play an essential role in extracting linguistic information from the brain. Their mediation is necessary for lifting objects, playing the piano, or doing any other activity. The fact that we do not become pigs or cows when we eat pork or beef is also due to genes. Genes are much more directly involved in the processes of day-to-day life than most people imagine.

Another fascinating feature is that, despite sharing common operating principles, the infinite possible combinations of genes ensure that no two entities will ever be identical. For any one child, there are seventy trillion possible combinations of genes. Therefore, the marriage of a beautiful woman with a brilliant man does not guarantee the birth of a handsome genius. A beautiful actress was once rumored to have proposed to George Bernard Shaw because she wanted a child with her beauty and his intelligence. The playwright, well-known for his sarcastic wit, responded, "And what if we have a child with your brains and my looks?"

You could also look at it this way: You exist because you just happened to be chosen from seventy trillion possibilities. That is how special you are.

But there is another piece of the picture that intrigues scientists like myself. Who wrote this amazing code in the first place? Human beings could not possibly have created the genetic code, but does that mean it just happened spontaneously? After all, the ingredients necessary for life abound in the natural world.

In my opinion, life cannot be the result of mere coincidence. If that were true, a car should be able to assemble itself spontaneously as long as all the requisite parts are gathered together in one spot. We know that this does not happen. Some greater being must be behind this, a force that transcends human understanding.

For over ten years, I have been calling this "Something Great." I do not know exactly what it is, but life, which functions exquisitely on the basis of an immense blueprint condensed within a tiny cell, is inconceivable without it.

Significant advances have been made in the field of life sciences that enable us to unravel the mysteries of life, one by one. Yet a whole team of Nobel Prize winners working together would still be unable to create a single bacterium. Creating life from scratch is beyond our capabilities. Despite our extraordinary technological feats, we must never forget that we owe our lives to nature's wonderful powers. Many people think "making babies" is quite simple, but this is an arrogant way of thinking. The only role we play is to create the opportunity for a life to be born and, once born, to give that life the nourishment it needs to grow. Children grow up naturally according to the finely crafted principles of life.

The Issue of Cloning

In response, some people may ask, "What about cloning?" Genetic technology has reached the point where we can make pure copies of higher animals. We have already produced sheep and monkey clones, and human embryos have already been duplicated in the lab. The birth of Dolly, the first cloned sheep, was indeed a momentous event. She was reproduced without the aid of a ram and from a mammary gland cell, not a reproductive cell, randomly extracted from an adult sheep. Until then, this was thought to be impossible. As the clones matured, we saw that they were besieged with health problems that shortened their lives, but they were indeed genetic copies of the original animal.

What significance does the successful cloning of higher animals have for the life sciences? It means that, in theory, a genetic copy of a human being could be produced from any cell taken from any part of a person's body. For example, a cell from Shigeo Nagashima, a famous Japanese ballplayer and coach, could be used to create multiple physically identical individuals.

In general, fertilized eggs have the ability to become an individual. This means that cell division will result in an independent organism. Similarly, a single cell taken from any leaf of a plant can become any other part, which is why a plant cutting placed in the ground will grow into a plant. Unlike plants, however, the fertilized eggs of animals lose this ability during the initial stage of cell division. Therefore, it was assumed that although lower organisms such as frogs could be cloned, it would never be possible to clone mammals. Scientists believed that once cells had differentiated, they could never return to their original state. The birth of Dolly completely shattered this assumption.

Dolly was made from a mammary gland cell extracted from an ewe. The function of mammary gland cells is to produce milk, and ordinarily they cannot work in any other way. In this case, the nucleus of the cell, which contains the DNA, was extracted, placed inside the egg cell of a different ewe, and implanted in a surrogate mother sheep. By applying external stimuli such as electric shocks to the unfertilized egg, the cell recovered the ability to undergo repeated cell division just like a fertilized egg.

Whereas a frog or mouse clone might have been harder for us to appreciate, the successful cloning of a sheep demonstrated the potential for applying this technology to humans. In the case of humans, cloning means we can produce a child from the genes of two men. It also means that a career woman who does not want to bother with a pregnancy could still have her own child. Technologically, such things are now within our reach.

Countries such as England, Germany, and Denmark foresaw this possibility early on and established laws banning the application of cloning technology to humans. Many other nations refuse to fund human clone research. The desire to implement these restraints is only natural, because once such technology has been created, it is difficult to rein it in. There is always a chance that someone will want a clone of him or herself and that someone capable of the technology will comply with this demand, regardless of any laws against it or the expense involved.

At the same time, the debate concerning cloning is riddled with misinformation. Although a frog clone appears to be exactly that—an identical copy—even if we were able to successfully produce a clone from the genes of a person, the child would never become an exact replica. Adolf Hitler, for example, became the man he was because he grew up in a specific environment and period of time. Were he born in a different time and place, he would certainly have led a very different life. Although physically identical, a Hitler clone would grow up to be entirely different in terms of personality.

Activate Beneficial Genes through "Genetic Thinking"

In Japan, there is a saying that "Illness comes from the mind." In other words, the way we think can make us sick or, conversely, help us get better. This, I believe, is exactly where genes come into play.

What we think affects how our genes work, and this results in either sickness or health. Some scientists even believe that our genes and the way they function determine whether or not we lead a happy life. This does not mean that human happiness is genetically predetermined at birth. Genes that govern happiness must exist latently within everyone.

The genes are just waiting to be switched on. What we must do is activate them and set them to work in a way that benefits our lives.

As far as we can tell, only about 5 to 10 percent of our genes are actually working; what the rest are doing remains unknown. In other words, it seems the majority of our genes are inactive. The fact that our psychological state can change the way our genes function may actually be because so many genes are dormant. Some of those genes we do not yet understand may respond strongly to our mental condition.

How, then, can we make our genes work in a way that makes us happy? The answer is by living each day to the fullest with a positive attitude. My hypothesis is that an enthusiastic approach to life leads to success and activates the genes that make us experience happiness. Life goes smoothly when we maintain a positive attitude and are full of enthusiasm and vitality. I call this living with your genes switched on, or "genetic thinking." This mental state activates good genes and deactivates bad genes. How it works is not yet fully understood, but the popular concept of "positive thinking" may be related to this principle. Many people who have changed the course of history exhibited a positive attitude.

I have also noticed that many Japanese scientists who were unproductive in Japan suddenly blossomed and achieved great things after moving to the United States. In this case, the change in environment appears to have activated their good genes. Like them, I also gained confidence and developed my foundation as a scientist when I moved to the United States in the early years of my career in biochemistry. There I transformed from a mediocre unknown to a successful scientist. Moving to a new country, of course, does not actually change a person's genes, and some people will insist that the change was due only to the new environment. However, exposure to a new environment can act as a trigger that switches on dormant genes. The United States is a country in which the "lone wolf" thrives. As in the case of Japanese pitcher Hideo Nomo, going to America has activated the genes of many Japanese who do not "fit in" at home. By working with a positive attitude in a new environment, they begin to produce results. And when they do, their achievements are recognized and they receive positive reinforcement. The opposite is also true. Scientists who see themselves as failures produce poor results. I cannot help feeling that their genes are just waiting to be activated.

Many people today seem to take a negative approach to life. From the perspective of their genes, this is detrimental. "I shouldn't overeat," "I mustn't drink too much," "I should quit smoking," "I've got to cut down on my salt intake," "I should lose weight," and "I should eat better" are examples of thoughts that do not work to activate beneficial genes. In other words, although the statements are statistically accurate, the belief that all of them apply to us personally can cause unnecessary stress, which in turn could have a negative impact on our genes. We do not know if these maxims hold true for each individual. There is no conclusive evidence, for example, that a body-fat ratio of over 25 percent is bad for everyone. While smoking is said to cause lung cancer, a significant percentage of heavy smokers do not get this disease. With further research on how our genes are affected, perhaps we would have a clearer picture. In the end, what is "good for you" depends on the individual. This may sound extreme, but if you really love smoking and do not bother other people, perhaps there is no need to quit. If you like a certain type of drink, enjoy it. If you crave a certain type of food, eat it. As long as it is not making you sick, you can enjoy it. It is even possible to live with cancer.

The important thing is to switch off as many harmful genes as possible and to activate helpful genes instead, getting them to work for you. The key to doing this is your way of thinking. I call this attitude "genetic thinking," and I have come to believe through my research and experience that it is an effective way to influence your genes and improve your life.

I

DECODING THE MYSTERY OF LIFE

Understanding Cells and Genes

To understand how you can influence your genes, let's begin by taking a look at the relationship between cells and genes. Our bodies are comprised of an enormous number of cells. The number of cells per kilogram of body weight is about one trillion; therefore, even a newborn baby has as many as three trillion cells. A person who weighs sixty kilograms (132 pounds) is made up of approximately sixty trillion cells. That number alone is mind-boggling, but even more astounding is the fact that, excluding a few exceptions, each cell contains the same genes.

The body is comprised of many different parts that look and function very differently. Hair, fingernails, and skin appear to have little in common. Yet they are all made up of cells that have basically the same structure and function. And furthermore, the genes that determine the functioning of those cells are also identical.

Let me give a simple explanation of cell structure. In the center of each cell is a nucleus covered by a membrane (see figure 1). Genes are located in the nucleus. If you traced your current existence back to its origins, you would find that you began as a single cell (a fertilized egg). One fertilized cell divides into two, two into four, four into eight, eight into sixteen, and so on. Somewhere during this process

Figure I
Cell structure

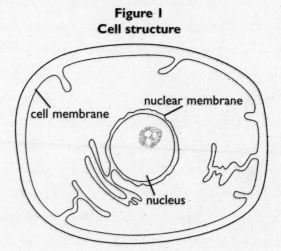

the cells begin to differentiate and specialize—some become the hands, others the legs, and others the brain or liver. They continue dividing within the mother's womb for nine months until at the time of birth a baby has about three trillion cells.

Of course, cell division continues after that, too, but the subject we are examining is the genes. The cell nucleus holds deoxyribonucleic acid (DNA), the substance that we call genes. DNA is made up of two spiral strands, the surfaces of which have molecules whose names are abbreviated as four letters: A, T, C, and G. This is our genetic code, and it is believed to contain all the information required for life. The nucleus of a single human cell contains three billion of these letters. Our lives literally depend on the vast amount of information encoded in our DNA.

The fact that the information contained in a single gene is identical to that contained in every one of the more than sixty trillion individual cells in our bodies means that any cell taken from any part could potentially be used to create another human being. A major question arises, however. If every cell in the human body contains the necessary information for living, why do the cells in our fingernails become only fingernails or the cells in our hair function only as hair? Theoretically, should it not be possible for a hair cell to suddenly decide it would like to change jobs for a day and be a heart cell or for a heart cell to decide to be a fingernail cell? As every cell contains a complete set of data, it inherently has this potential.

In reality, however, this never happens. It is believed that the genes in the cells of our fingernails have been programmed or switched on to "nail mode," while all other possibilities have been deactivated or switched off. We still do not understand the details of how this mechanism works, but somewhere during the process of cell division from a fertilized egg, our cells come to some form of agreement among themselves concerning the division of labor. Thereafter each cell faithfully follows those rules.

The On/Off Mechanism

Genes in each cell nucleus store a vast amount of information, including instructions concerning how to function in certain situations and when to stop functioning. Geneticists refer to these instructions as the on/off mechanism. When do genes, which seem almost infinite in number, switch on or off?

Some are activated after the passage of a specific period of time. Those that govern the growth of breasts or facial hair during puberty are a good example. When children reach this stage, previously dormant genes governing hormone production switch on. As a result, boys become more masculine and girls become more feminine.

It is thought that both the surrounding environment and our emotional or mental condition can accelerate or retard this process. This interrelationship is not yet clearly understood. Many scientists are conducting research on how genes affect a person's character, disposition, and behavior, while my own research focuses on how psychological factors affect genes. For the time being, the idea that psychological action is deeply related to the on/off mechanism in our genes is only one hypothesis, but I believe that it will be verified with ongoing research.

The fact that this on/off mechanism exists is no longer hypothesis. About forty years ago, François Jacob and Jacques Monod, two scientists working for the Pasteur Institute in Paris, discovered a function very similar to an on/off switch during an experiment on *E. coli*, a bacteria that usually lives in the intestines.

E. coli bacteria consume primarily glucose. When both lactose and glucose are present, the bacteria will exclusively choose the latter. In this experiment, the bacteria did not respond at all to lactose when it was provided along with glucose. In the next step, they were given lactose only. At first, the bacteria ate nothing, but within a short space of time they began consuming lactose and started to multiply.

To a layperson, this may seem obvious, but to a scientist it is a revelation. From their experiment, Jacob and Monod hoped to determine whether or not the ability to digest lactose was acquired only after the bacteria began receiving lactose or whether it was present from the beginning. After much investigation, they concluded that it already existed and was not newly acquired. In other words, *E. coli* bacteria inherently possess the ability to produce lactose-degrading enzymes (lactase). When glucose was available, the enzyme-producing gene was switched off, but when only lactose was available and the bacteria had to digest it in order to survive, the gene was activated. It was not that a nonexistent ability spontaneously emerged but rather that an existing ability lay dormant. This represented a tremendous breakthrough in our understanding of genes.

What Code Is Written in Our Genes?

Let me give you a basic outline of how our genes work. The wealth of information that genes contain is encoded on DNA within our cells, and I am not speaking metaphorically.

About fifty years ago, a momentous discovery was made: All living things use the same genetic code. This means that everything—whether mold, *E. coli* bacteria, plants, animals, or human beings—functions according to the same principle. The basic unit of all living creatures is the cell; genes determine cell function; and genes operate according to common principles. This is evidence that all living things originated from a single cell. Perhaps this is why so many people feel calm and peaceful when surrounded by plants and trees or why they feel a close affinity to animals such as dogs or cats. As everything originally sprang from the same source, we are all related.

This knowledge subsequently helped scientists to unravel many of the mysteries of life. We have even succeeded in decoding human genes. This, in turn, has led to further unexpected discoveries. We now know, for example, just how small our genes are. The human genetic code, comprised of over three billion "chemical letters," is all stored within microscopic strands that weigh only one 200-billionth of a gram and are only 1/500,000 millimeter wide—and yet, if they were stretched out, they would be about three meters long.

If you could slice a one-millimeter diameter wire lengthwise into one-hundredths, the result would be strands so delicate they would shatter with a puff of air, yet each would still be five thousand times thicker than a strand of DNA. To help you understand just how tiny that is, imagine that you could collect all the DNA from the world's population of six billion people. It would weigh only as much as a single grain of rice. The world of our genes is infinitesimally small.

Let me add a few more pertinent facts. Genes are the blueprint of life, the key element that makes it possible to transmit life from one generation to the next, and cells are the basic unit of all living things. As shown in figure 2, DNA has at its foundation a long, double-stranded chain of a complex combination of simple sugars and phosphates. Characteristically, the two strands form a right-handed helical spiral resembling a ladder that is called a "double helix." These strands have connecting "rungs" at regular intervals made of four chemicals.

All genetic information in any organism is written on this double helix at points corresponding to the "rungs" of the

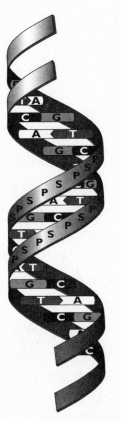

Figure 2
Gene (DNA) structure

DNA is a combination of four chemicals—adenine, thymine, cytosine, and guanine—plus two strands made of sugars and phosphates.

Adenine pairs with thymine and cytosine with guanine to form base pairs—the "rungs" of the twisted ladder known as DNA.

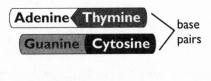

> base pairs

P=phosphate
S=sugar(deoxyribose)

ladder using four "chemical letters"—A, T, C, and G, which stand for the chemicals adenine, thymine, cytosine, and guanine. The four chemicals are paired—adenine with thymine and cytosine with guanine—and these pairs join the two sugar-phosphate strands together to make the double-helix shape. This is DNA, our genes. The information contained in our genes, which is known as genetic information, is equivalent to three billion of these chemical letters, and if printed in book form, it would amount to three thousand volumes each a thousand pages long.

That the structure of such a complex living organism as a human being is determined by information encoded in only four chemical letters is amazing. Even more amazing is the fact that the basic genetic structure of all living things, from the tiniest microbes to highly complex animals, is identical. In fact, over 90 percent of human genes are identical to plant genes. Single-cell organisms such as mold or *E. coli* bacteria operate according to the same basic principles as human beings, which are comprised of more than sixty trillion cells. Most amazing of all, however, is the microscopic size of the DNA containing this huge volume of genetic information.

DNA Decoding Chart Identifies Proteins

I was in a state of perpetual amazement when I began to study genes. No matter which aspect of the DNA I looked at, I was struck by the miraculous nature of life. How on earth, I wondered, could such a minute yet precise blueprint for life have been created? I was constantly pondering such questions.

The structure of DNA was discovered in 1953, and since then research aimed at deciphering the mysteries of life has progressed so rapidly that we can now read the blueprint written on the DNA—the genetic code of bacteria, animals, and even humans.

But what exactly is this code and how do we read it? The genetic code is the set of instructions for making proteins. Protein along with water is one of the most important substances in our bodies. It is not only a structural element but is also found in the enzymes essential to the chemical reactions that take place inside us. In other words, protein is the foundation of the phenomenon we call life.

Proteins are made from twenty different kinds of amino acids. The type of protein that is made depends on how those amino acids are combined. DNA provides the instructions that govern the manufacture and order of the twenty types of amino acids. The chemical pairs that make up the rungs of the ladder combine in three-letter "words." Because adenine (A) is always paired with thymine (T), and cytosine (C) with guanine (G)—even though sometimes they "flip" from AT to TA or CG to GC—we refer to the "words" by only the first letter of the pair. In the three-letter "word" ATG, for example, A comes first, T second, and G third as we climb the rungs of the ladder. According to the decoding chart in figure 3, this combination represents the instructions for making the amino acid methionine. Identifying a specific amino acid from triplets of the chemical bases A, T, C, and G is known as reading the genetic code.

The four chemical letters A, T, C, and G are like the alphabet, and the three-letter amino acid identifications (triplets) comprised of these are like the words in a dictionary. The amino acid glutamine, for example, is expressed as the "word" GAA or GAG. With the chart in figure 3, we can theoretically decode the genetic information of every living creature.

To make it simpler, imagine that each cell contains a library. When a cell wants to do something, it goes to the library; opens a book; learns when, what, and how to do it; and then begins implementing the task exactly as learned. The book is our genes or DNA, and the content of the book is genetic information.

Figure 3
DNA decoding chart

First letter	Second letter				Third letter
	T	C	A	G	
T	phenylalanine	serine	tyrosine	cysteine	T
	phenylalanine	serine	tyrosine	cysteine	C
	leucine	serine	stop	stop	A
	leucine	serine	stop	tryptophan	G
C	leucine	proline	histidine	arginine	T
	leucine	proline	histidine	arginine	C
	leucine	proline	glutamine	arginine	A
	leucine	proline	glutamine	arginine	G
A	isoleucine	threonine	asparagine	serine	T
	isoleucine	threonine	asparagine	serine	C
	isoleucine	threonine	lysine	arginine	A
	methionine (start)	threonine	lysine	arginine	G
G	valine	alanine	aspartic acid	glycine	T
	valine	alanine	aspartic acid	glycine	C
	valine	alanine	glutamic acid	glycine	A
	valine (start)	alanine	glutamic acid	glycine	G

A triplet selected from the four bases (T, C, A, and G) specifies one amino acid.

But a book is just a book. No matter how delicious a recipe it contains, it cannot satisfy our hunger. Unless we follow the recipe to make the dish, it remains a picture in a book. This is where the cook, messenger RNA (ribonucleic acid), comes in. Messenger RNA goes to the DNA, copies the information written there in a process known as "transcribing," and makes proteins based on this copy using amino acids as the ingredients. The proteins, then, do the work of the cell.

Genes That Regulate the On/Off Switch

In order to understand the on/off mechanism, you must first be acquainted with the important role of proteins. Proteins are the most fundamental component of every living creature. Recognized as an essential part of our diet, they are classified in the field of nutritional science as one of three macronutrients along with fats and carbohydrates. What are the relationships between these three?

Think of a house. The foundation, building materials, and furniture—everything that has a definable shape—are all made of proteins. Fats fill in the gaps in the building materials and protect the structure. Carbohydrates provide energy, just like electricity and gas.

To live means to reside in this house. Even if we have a supply of electricity and gas and the insulation material required to fill in the gaps, these alone do not make a house. First we need the stones for the foundation and the lumber for the posts, beams, flooring, and wall materials. It is proteins that fulfill this role. Proteins make up not only the framework, floors, and walls of the house but also the appliances such as the vacuum cleaner and the washing machine as well as the cooking pots, utensils, and dishes.

It is our genes that decide what kind of protein and how much to make. The ingredients used to make them are amino acids. Our bodies can manufacture twelve of the twenty types of amino acids. The other eight must be obtained from external sources. These eight are known as essential amino acids. A protein is a particular combination of amino acids. The amino acid composition of the meat of pigs or cows, for example, is different from that of humans. This is why we must first break down the pork or beef we eat into amino acids and then reconstitute it into the necessary proteins to make our bones, muscles, skin, and organs, following instructions given by our genes. Our bodies also secrete important hormones and enzymes. Almost all of these are proteins too.

Proteins are also an important part of the genetic on/off mechanism. To illustrate how this mechanism works so you can see how it is applied to waking up your own dormant genes, let me use the previously described experiment with *E. coli* bacteria and lactose conducted by Jacob and Monod. Figure 4 depicts the change that occurred when *E. coli* bacteria switched from eating glucose to lactose. The upper half of the figure (A) shows the bacteria when it is being supplied with glucose. When glucose is present, a special inhibiting protein (repressor) produced by a regulator gene is attached to the part of the gene that begins reading genetic information (operator), preventing it from reading the genetic information beyond that point. In other words, the gene is switched off.

This is similar to the way stores wrap books in plastic to prevent customers from reading them prior to purchase. Even if you find the book you have been looking for, you cannot open it and read it unless you remove the plastic wrapper. The book is there but it cannot be read, just like the lactose-degrading instructions in the bacteria genes described above. But when glucose is no longer available and the bacteria are forced to digest lactose in order to obtain nutrients, the genes change as shown in the lower half of the figure (B), enabling them to read the information. In (B), the repressor combines with lactose so that it no longer inhibits the operator, allowing

Figure 4
The genetic on/off mechanism

A. GLUCOSE AVAILABLE

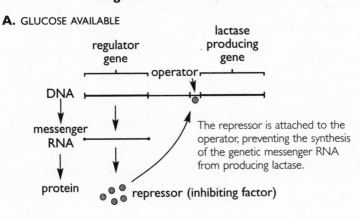

The repressor is attached to the operator, preventing the synthesis of the genetic messenger RNA from producing lactase.

repressor (inhibiting factor)

B. LACTOSE AVAILABLE,
GLUCOSE ABSENT

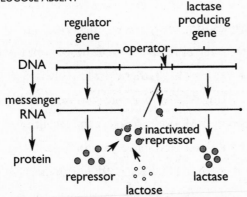

it to begin producing lactase. In our analogy of the bookstore, the plastic wrapper has been removed from the "book" so that it can be read, and the gene is now switched on.

In other words, although genes come equipped with a vast amount of information, not all of it is being used. Genes in the nucleus are transcribed to each messenger RNA when needed. The messenger RNA in cells are translated instantly to proteins and enzymes, which are the most important substances for the activity of cells. At the same time, however, they prevent unnecessary information from being read. This function operates just like the switch on an electrical appliance, which is why geneticists began calling it the on/off mechanism. The glucose/lactose experiment proved for the first time that genes inherently possess this function.

The fact that certain capacities do not spontaneously materialize from nothing but rather exist latently in our genes was an epoch-making discovery. In order to explain this phenomenon, Jacob and Monod proposed the hypothesis that there are structural genes that make protein as well as regulator genes that turn the gene on or off. This hypothesis was subsequently proved and is known as the Operon Theory. Jacob and Monod along with André M. Lwoff were awarded the Nobel Prize in Physiology or Medicine in 1965 in recognition of their scientific achievement. Thanks to their pioneering work, we are all the closer to analyzing the potential of genes and, in the case of my work, how we can activate our beneficial genes to make them work for us.

Chemical Reactions Happen Constantly within Us

Many people are under the misapprehension that genes are merely passed on from parent to child and do not have much to do with daily living. This is far from true. Genes are active every minute, every second of our lives, and if they stopped working, we would die instantly.

Everything that occurs in our bodies is the result of chemical reactions. It may seem uninspiring to describe life as a chemical reaction, but this is scientifically accurate. A good example is the superhuman strength that people sometimes experience in times of crisis. I am sure that you have heard of people being able to lift impossibly heavy objects during an emergency such as an accident or fire. Someone who is normally capable of lifting a maximum of only fifty kilograms will suddenly lift one hundred kilograms. People tend to attribute this to psychological reasons. They claim that anything is possible if your desire to achieve it is strong enough. But without some form of chemical reaction to make it possible, you cannot do anything, no matter how desperately you want to.

The first requirement is energy. In an emergency, genes that up to now have ordered the production of only enough energy to lift fifty kilograms command the cell to produce double the energy. In fact, every life process is the result of chemical reactions that are intended to cope with a particular situation. This is what "living" means.

Chemical manufacturing plants also produce chemical reactions. From a biochemical perspective, these reactions are theoretically similar to those that constitute the process we call living. There is, however, a decisive difference between the chemical reactions that take place in our bodies and those that take place in chemical-manufacturing plants.

Chemical reactions in manufacturing plants can occur only under extreme conditions such as exposure to high temperature, high pressure, high acidity, or high alkalinity. The chemical reactions that take place within living cells, on the other hand, occur in a very ordinary environment at normal body temperature and pressure and in a neutral state. It is enzymes that make this possible. Although they are not the principal actors in the process, enzymes function as catalysts, acting upon specific substances to make chemical reactions occur smoothly. Thousands of such chemical reactions are occurring systematically and very rapidly within every cell, each of which weighs only about one-billionth of a gram, and enzymes play a crucial role in this process.

In the case of hypertension, the enzyme renin is considered to increase hypertension. In fact, it does not do this itself but instead produces the hormone angiotensin, which raises blood pressure. Thus, it is really controlling hypertension from behind the scenes, using a subordinate hormone to do the work.

One striking characteristic of enzymes is the fact that they bond only with specific substances. Just like a lock and key, the counterpart of any enzyme is predetermined— enzyme A bonds with *a*, enzyme B bonds with *b*, and so on. Enzymes are able to select their counterpart with absolute precision, and this makes it possible for several thousands of chemical reactions to occur simultaneously within each cell.

Another feature of enzymes is speed. Let's assume, for example, that a cell needs to produce a certain substance. If it already has the materials, the presence of an enzyme makes it possible to manufacture the necessary substance up to ten billion times faster than normal. Starch by itself will remain starch even after the passage of one year, changing only gradually. Yet when ingested, it undergoes numerous chemical reactions within just a few hours to produce energy. Once inside our bodies, chemical reactions take place at a speed unimaginable in the external world.

Some people are under the false impression that after our bodies have reached adulthood, not much change takes place. After all, once we have stopped growing, our height and weight usually remain fairly constant. But contrary to outward appearances, replacement and change are occurring at a tremendous rate. An adult's red blood cells disintegrate at a rate of several hundred billion per day only to be replaced by the same amount of new blood cells. Proteins in our kidneys, liver, and heart are degenerating and regenerating at immeasurable speed. This is known as metabolic turnover, and it happens much more rapidly than we could ever imagine. The chemical reactions of synthesis and disintegration are occurring as programmed at lightning speed within our cells thanks to enzymes.

Enzymes, with their almost magical powers, are controlled by receptors, which are controlled by genes. Therefore, by influencing our genes, we can indirectly control enzymes. Some of the miraculous things that happen around us may actually be caused by the effects of the mind on a person's genes, which in turn stimulate high-speed chemical reactions. Although this is difficult to prove directly, much circumstantial evidence supports it.

Two examples come to mind. When I was a student, some high-spirited Buddhist monks undergoing rigorous ascetic training used to come down from their mountain retreat night after night to carouse in the entertainment districts, returning at dawn in order to perform their duties. Some had such stamina that they could keep this up for several days in a row. The desire to play was enough to prevent them from feeling any fatigue the next day. Similarly, some assistants in my lab seem lethargic and fail to respond to any urging from me to work harder. But when their research is approaching an international breakthrough and comes under the spotlight, they will work all night long without a single complaint. Once they are motivated, they no longer feel tired even though they lack sufficient sleep.

When we have to meet someone we really do not want to see, our feet feel like lead and move reluctantly or even come to a halt. On the other hand, when we are on our way to meet someone we really like and want to see, our feet feel so light we could almost fly.

These physical manifestations of our emotions would be impossible without the action of several different enzymes, the production speed of which is controlled by genes. Therefore, these phenomena must also be caused by the genetic on/off mechanism.

Take the case of a person's hair turning white overnight after psychological trauma. Genes unceasingly manufacture the protein that comprises our hair. Such an abrupt and dramatic change must mean that the genes supporting normal hair growth have been turned off or that those which would normally cause aging in the future have been activated early. Genes are clearly behind many of our daily phenomena.

In the next chapter, we'll take a closer look at physical manifestations of our psychological state and see ways we can begin to positively influence our genes.

II

ACTIVATE YOUR GENES

The Role of Positive Thinking in
Awakening Beneficial Genes

Obviously, some genes are better activated while others are better deactivated. Ideally, harmful genes should be switched off and beneficial genes switched on. Positive thinking, I believe, is an important key to this.

The concepts of positive and negative thinking are now so familiar to us that the phrase "think positively" has become part of our daily lexicon. In life, however, both good and bad things happen. It is not always easy to stay positive when things go wrong, and some people may even wonder why there is so much hype about it. To help clarify the difference between the two, let's compare positive and negative thinking from the perspective of entropy.

What happens when you add a single drop of ink to a sink full of water? The ink immediately begins to disperse. Why doesn't it gather in one spot instead? This phenomenon has profound implications. In the physical world, organized matter is believed to move naturally toward disorganization or decay. This is known as the law of increasing entropy. Far from being limited to ink, increasing entropy is recognized as a general rule that applies to the material world as a whole. As we also are made of matter, we are automatically subject to this law. From the moment of birth, we move toward destruction and death. The only conceivable reason for this is the existence of genes inside us that naturally gravitate toward disorganization. The truth is that our bodies come equipped with a program for cell death.

If these genes suddenly began working to their fullest extent, it would mean instant death because the genes would wear out. Normally, however, our genes are working to keep us alive and to prevent increasing entropy. In other words, the act of living can be seen as taking the processes that naturally gravitate toward death and decay and directing them toward order. This is known as entropy reduction. For example, a dictionary as a book has a specific function. But what if you ripped out all the pages and scattered them about the room? The total volume of material that comprised the book has not decreased at all, but it no longer serves the function of a dictionary. This is what entropy increase looks like. But if you gathered all the scattered pages and painstakingly glued them back together, the dictionary would return to its original state. This is entropy reduction.

Genes and the enzymes produced under their direction play an important role in reducing entropy. When we eat pork, for example, the protein is first broken down into the component amino acids and these are then recombined into human protein by enzymes under the direction of genes. The decomposition represents an increase of entropy while the synthesis represents a reduction of entropy.

If we apply the principle of entropy to the concept of positive and negative thinking, it is appropriate to consider that positive thinking leads to entropy reduction while negative thinking leads to entropy increase. You'll see why this is so in the diabetes/laughter study that follows. If positive thinking does in fact lead to entropy reduction, as my own experience has led me to believe, then the choice to think positively or negatively is quite different from choosing to eat sweet or spicy foods. In the latter case, it is merely a matter of personal taste and does not really make a difference. As long as we do not overindulge, we can have both nutrition and pleasure. With negative or positive thinking, however, the option we choose will most certainly have consequences. There is no question about which is better. Positive thinking will cause our genes to work hard to reduce entropy, while negative thinking will accelerate entropy increase.

An experiment that I conducted in 2003 resulted in scientific evidence corroborating the beneficial impact of positive thinking on genes. Based on the fact that genes are switched on or off by physical or chemical factors, I proposed the hypothesis that mental factors are also involved in switching genes on or off. To be more specific, positive factors, such as joy, excitement, belief, and prayer, upregulate—or activate—transcripts of valuable genes, while negative factors, such as anxiety, stress, sadness, fear, and pain, downregulate—or deactivate—transcripts of valuable genes.

To test my hypothesis, we joined forces with Japan's entertainment business giant Yoshimoto Kogyo Co. to study the effect of laughter (an indicator of positive emotion) on gene expression. We specifically focused on how laughter would affect blood-glucose levels in people with type 2 diabetes. In our study, we measured test subjects' fasting blood glucose (FBG), after which they listened to either a humorless lecture or a comedy show. Then they were served a meal, after which we tested their post-prandial (after-meal) blood glucose (PPBG). In the first experiment, those who watched the lecture had a 123 mg/dL increase in blood-glucose levels, while those who watched the comedy show only a 77 mg/dL increase. We repeated the experiment, and once again, those who watched the comedy had a significantly smaller increase in PPBG than those who didn't.

Laughter, the study showed, has a beneficial effect on blood-glucose levels. We found that twenty-three genes were activated from laughing. In addition, one gene that we identified as being activated by laughter, dopamine D4 receptor gene (DRD4), is linked to inhibition of the enzyme adenylyl cyciase, which plays a role in increasing blood-glucose levels. This result could prove to be useful in maintaining blood-glucose levels in patients with diabetes. But the implications went far beyond than that: for the first time it was proven that positive emotion can flip the genetic switch. These findings were published in the journal *Diabetes Care* in May 2003 and the journal *Psychotherapy and Psychosomatics* in 2006 and were reported by Reuters around the world.

Seeing the Positive

Anecdotal evidence also points to the tangible effects of a positive or negative mental state. Psychological trauma, as I mentioned previously, can switch on a gene that causes all our hair to turn gray overnight, a process that would normally take several decades. But what amazing things could be done if we could use this same gene in a positive direction? The problem, of course, is how. If trauma is the effect of a negative mental shock, then it makes sense that the opposite, something that makes us very happy, should activate positive genes. As our genes are working every minute, every second without rest, we would have to keep our mind constantly focused on that feeling of happiness. The secret to doing this is to practice positive thinking.

We must be particularly conscious of positive thinking during times of difficulty and suffering, because this is when positive thinking is really necessary. It is far easier to think positively when things are going well. The true test is how positively we can think when we are confronted with a difficult situation. In fact, we probably do not even need to concern ourselves with positive thinking when things are going smoothly.

Speaking from personal experience, scientists frequently confront difficult situations during long research projects. It is not unusual to be assailed by a sense of failure and hopelessness. The point is to look for ways to avoid becoming discouraged at such times.

I have one technique that works for me. I remind myself that any situation in life has two sides: its good points as well as its bad points. It just depends on your interpretation. Take illness, for example. When you get sick, it is easy to focus on the negative: it prevents you from working and causes financial strain. At the same time, though, it can have positive effects such as helping you appreciate the special people in your life or giving you time to think of ideas that were obstructed by a busy work schedule. You have probably heard at least a few stories of how a severe illness turned someone's life toward a positive direction. The trick is to take a broader perspective and to trust and believe that illness will help you develop in a constructive way. We need to see the bigger picture and endeavor to see the positive in everything that happens to us in life.

If you think that this is impossible, your response actually reflects one of modern man's shortcomings. Science excels at rational thinking. Because science has advanced so dramatically, people have fallen into the habit of trying to rationalize everything. Scientific thought is based on logical positivism, but this approach weakens our receptivity to those things that transcend reason—to the invisible realm. Rationality is important up to a certain point, but not everything in this world is rational.

Genes are the ultimate example. Cells and the genes inside them are part of a microscopic world invisible to the naked eye. Moreover, of the enormous number of genes in our bodies, only 5 to 10 percent is functioning at one time. Scientists have no idea what the rest are doing. Perhaps the remaining genes contain the history of our evolution, or maybe they store the potential for future development. We do not yet know what their significance is. I believe that the genetic on/off mechanism is related to this unknown portion. If we focus solely on the rational, we can perceive only part of our reality. To transcend rationality does not mean to enter an irrational world but rather to acknowledge those aspects that cannot be explained by conventional wisdom or current science when we make decisions. This approach can help us grasp the overall picture even if it is a little fuzzy. Positive thinking is one way to develop such a perspective.

The Mind Has Tremendous Influence on the Individual

The power of positive thinking is often demonstrated when a person becomes ill. There are many aspects of the natural healing mechanism that we still do not understand, but one thing is clear to me: Genes play an indispensable role. If, for example, a doctor tells a patient that he or she has cancer, even a very emotionally stable person will feel depressed. Until recently, it was common practice in Japan for doctors not to tell their patients they had cancer, partly because treatment methods were as yet undeveloped but also because patients clearly found such information traumatic. Informed consent has become the norm not only because treatment methods have greatly advanced but also because scientists now recognize the validity of the proverb "Illness comes from the mind."

Even so, some scientists may reject as unscientific any claim that the mind governs genetic functioning and self-healing because of the logical positivism on which scientific research is based. At the same time, however, this claim cannot be dismissed as false merely because contemporary science is unable to prove it. After all, many errors have been made in the history of science. Moreover, many things we know to be beneficial in our daily lives, such as the effects of meditation or prayer, cannot be scientifically proven.

The concept of self-healing has existed since ancient times. The idea is that the body heals itself, but another way to express this, I feel, is that the genes command the body to heal. In other words, the body comes equipped with a latent healing program. Nothing can happen inside the body unless it is already written in our genes. Fortunately for us, there are countless options from which our genes can choose; the large percentage of each gene that is unused holds the possibility for self-healing. So what is currently being expressed by our genes is not the final say. Good genes can switch on and harmful genes can turn off.

We all have genes that can potentially cause illness and, at the same time, genes that can suppress illness. Both cancer-causing and cancer-inhibiting genes have been found; when they exist together, they maintain a balance. Other illnesses are the same. The important point is balance. Although we cannot actually trace all the changes that occur inside the body, imagine that a cancer gene has switched on inside you and begins producing cancer cells. As soon as it does, the gene responsible for inhibiting and eliminating such cells begins to work, keeping you healthy. Your body is in a state of equilibrium. But once that balance is upset, the disease begins to spread rapidly.

Cancer is difficult to treat due to the sheer number of cancer-causing factors. Until recently, external factors in the environment were thought to be the trigger, including diet, smoking, drinking contaminated water, and chemical additives in food, all of which were labeled "dangerous." Although these substances may indeed pose risks, genetic research has clearly shown that their influence varies greatly depending on the individual. This is most likely due to the uniqueness of each individual's genetic makeup.

My research leads me to believe that the reason people who have never smoked even one cigarette still get lung cancer is because they carry inside them cancer-promoting genes. When this factor is combined with environmental factors to which everyone is equally exposed, it causes acceleration of the cancer-promoting function. Although I do not know exactly how this mechanism works, it is likely behind the cause of many illnesses.

Environmental factors are a crucial variable in whether harmful genes are switched off. Even if two people had exactly the same genes—identical twins—and one became ill, the other may not become sick because each was exposed to different environmental factors. In a healthy person, the genes that cause the illness are switched off, but at a certain point they may be activated. Scientists are currently making progress in cataloging genetic variations that are linked to common diseases such as heart disease and lung cancer. With further research, we will be able to predict more accurately when genes will activate and how to switch them off. When we do, I am certain that the impact of environment on this on/off mechanism will be better understood.

Today few deny the relationship between the mind and the body, but many consider only the external or physical environment—such as air, noise, and water pollution—when they hear the term "environmental factors." But I feel that the environment includes the psychological impact of information concerning the physical environment. The mind is not separate from the environment.

In an interview, Shigeo Nozawa, originator of the hydroponic agricultural method, which I will talk about more in chapter 6, explained this idea as follows: "In the case of human beings, the state of a person's mind itself is their environment. The state of being happy or healthy originates in the mind. People may assume that a certain type of environment is ideal, but actually any environment that an individual perceives to be good is beneficial because the environment and the life processes of the individual mutually interact. There is no absolute good or bad environment." I agree with this statement wholeheartedly.

The mind has a tremendous influence on the individual. Just as Nozawa said, illness, failing to pass an exam, or losing one's job, when interpreted positively, can all be accepted with gratitude. These experiences help us deepen our understanding of life and make us more sympathetic to the suffering of other people. They may even launch us toward a bright new future. You most likely have endured times, as I have, when you thought you had failed at a goal but it turned out that you had not failed at all. I am convinced from my own experience that what Nozawa said is true: The state of being happy or healthy originates in the mind.

There is one way to deactivate harmful genes and activate good ones that is accessible to everyone regardless of their environment or circumstances: changing one's mental attitude. It's impossible to deny that mental attitude, both positive and negative, has a major effect on our health. I suspect that the interaction between the mind and the body is even greater than previously thought. Although the relationship between our genes and psychological action remains unclear, genes hold the key to understanding the body's natural healing mechanism.

Our Genes Act Before We Think

There is another point I would like to mention in regard to the human thought process. Most people believe that the brain plays the most important role in governing action. It is in fact the cells and the network connecting the cells that is doing all the work, and it is the genes that direct the cells. Brain function depends on the information contained in the brain cells. In that sense, genes act as the body's main control panel. If it is possible for us to control the on/off mechanism of our genes, then we need to get to know our genes much better. We should pay attention to the messages we send them. It might even help to greet our genes with, "Hi, there! Glad to see you're in such good shape today. You're doing a great job." Since we carry on a constant dialogue with ourselves anyway, it can't hurt to direct positive thoughts to our genes.

Without even realizing it, we continuously engage in conversation with ourselves. When we are worried, we follow a script that is written from a negative perspective. On the other hand, going out on a sunny morning may cause us to exclaim, "What a beautiful day! I feel great!" At that moment our cells are benefiting. We do not need to register the sunshine visually first and wait for the brain to convey this information to the rest of our body. As soon as we step outside, our cells instantly respond to the pleasant weather and are activated. Although cells follow instructions from the brain, at the same time, they are independent individual organisms. This is an important point when considering the on/off mechanism.

In reality, we all go through periods in our lives when we are not healthy or bursting with energy. You may run into problems at work or have difficulties in your relationships with others. At such times it is hard not to feel depressed. How can you extricate yourself from feeling depressed when this happens? By turning on those genes that give you energy. You can learn how to do this by drawing on the wisdom you have gained through living. One method I recommend from my own experience is to let yourself be inspired. If nothing inspires you at the moment, think back to a time when you were deeply moved.

Inspiration is a combination of joy and pleasant excitement. Scientists feel this strongly when they have just finished a research project. The excitement and joy I feel when I have written a good paper is priceless. I have actually slept all night with a newly completed manuscript wrapped in my arms.

Another thing that inspires me is my work with genes. To work with genes is to be involved with the mechanism of life and to be frequently exposed to its wonders. This is a profoundly moving experience.

I believe that when we are inspired, our genes never move in an adverse direction. I am sure that I have my share of undesirable genes, but when I am moved and inspired, those genes are deactivated and in their stead beneficial genes are activated. Call it intuition or a scientist's hypothesis, but when I feel inspired, I can feel the wellness spreading all the way to my cells.

What inspires people will vary. For some it may be pursuing their passion through their career, spending time with their children, or enjoying the thrill of mountain climbing, gardening, or creating art. Something that fails to touch one person may profoundly move another. As an example, let me introduce Ko Hirasawa, one of my mentors and a former president of Kyoto University. When I was still a student, Hirasawa told me a story that I have never forgotten. When he joined the Kyoto University Medical Department, Hirasawa studied so hard that he slept only about four hours a night, Napoleon-style. As a result, he had a severe nervous breakdown and had to return to his hometown to recuperate. When he was wandering through a snowy field one day, he heard a voice reciting the *Heiligenstädter testament* in German, a statement written by Beethoven at the age of twenty-eight. An avid student, Hirasawa had read Beethoven's biography in the original German while pursuing his medical studies.

When Beethoven lost his hearing, he contemplated suicide and went so far as to write his will. After a long internal debate, however, he finally decided to live. He wrote the

Heiligenstädter testament at that time as an expression of this determination. In it, he states, "Perhaps I shall get better, perhaps not; I am ready.... Forced to become a philosopher already in my twenty-eighth year ... oh it is not easy, and for the artist much more difficult than for anyone else."

These words struck Hirasawa like a bolt of lightning. "My suffering is nothing! Beethoven overcame deafness, a fatal disability for a musician. I may not have great talent, but I do have a normal, healthy body, so how can I complain? I'll show everyone that I can overcome this!" Hirasawa was deeply moved, and at that moment his neurosis was cured. The frequent auditory and visual hallucinations he had suffered after his nervous breakdown disappeared. What could have instantaneously cured such a severe condition? I think the profound emotion he experienced may have activated those genes that cause healing and vitality. His experience can inspire us as well.

The Key to Youth and Longevity

There is one method of interacting with your genes that I highly recommend for your longevity: being profoundly moved and deeply inspired on a regular basis.

To live, we must discharge various substances from our body daily, including stool, urine, sweat, and mucous. We also need to trim our hair and nails periodically. Without excretion and secretion, we could not survive for a single day. You may have noticed that all the substances listed above share one common feature: as soon as they are discharged, they become waste products. When they are inside, we do not view them as particularly dirty, but once they leave our bodies, we view them as unclean. But I have noticed that there is one substance we excrete that does not inspire disgust: tears.

Tears are also a bodily waste, but no one regards them with the same aversion as they do other types of waste. Hypocrites regard tears not as a waste product but rather as a bodily fluid derived from the brain. The theologian Tetsuo Yamaori pointed out to me that tears touch the hearts of others. The sparkle of tears draws out our emotions.

People often cry when they are deeply moved. Although strong emotion brings tears to our eyes, physiologically it is our genes that make this happen, which is an indication of how the mind influences our genes. Being moved to tears feels good, and even when we are sad, a good cry can be a tremendous release that leaves us feeling better. Feeling good is an indication, I believe, that our good genes have been activated. Many elderly people cite deep emotion as a key to longevity. The same is true of people who appear more youthful than their years. Experiencing profound emotion can make us live longer and keep us young, and once again, our genes must be involved. Although I do not understand how emotions are inspired within our minds, I do know that when I am moved to tears, my heart feels cleansed and there is no place in it for hatred or resentment. To live a long, full life, I highly recommend pursuing activities and relationships that inspire sincere emotion from the depths of your heart.

What Is Not Written in Our Genes Cannot Be Done

Some people claim that human potential is infinite. They think that if a person tries hard enough, he or she can do or become anything. Others insist that just as a tadpole must become a frog, our limitations are predetermined from birth. These conflicting viewpoints often cause heated debate. The fact is that we cannot do anything unless it is already programmed in our genes. In that sense, human potential and capacity is indeed limited.

If I suddenly exhibit traits that were not evident before—for example, if I suddenly become more hardworking, persistent, or peaceful—this is simply the emergence of inherent traits that had not yet surfaced. Either the genetic switch for those abilities has been turned on or the genetic switch for such traits as laziness or pleasure seeking has been turned off for some reason. A person's capacity is entirely encoded in their genes.

But we must remember that only 5 or at most 10 percent of the genes in the whole human genome, or set of genetic information, are believed to be functioning at any given time while the rest remain dormant. In other words, although the genome inside each cell contain three billion pieces of genetic information encoded in the letters A, T, C, and G, the vast majority of genes are not in use. Accordingly, although I have said that human potential is limited, my definition of "limited" differs dramatically from the conventional interpretation. First, for everything, there is always a possibility. In that sense, the perspective that human potential is limitless is not mistaken. Whatever our brains believe to be possible is indeed possible, and whatever we are not thinking about is outside the realm of both possibility and impossibility. The airplane, for example, was invented because someone thought, "I want to fly like a bird." Although, scientifically speaking, human potential is limited, we do not need to be conscious of this limit because the information written in our genes far exceeds anything we could ever imagine.

At this time, the human limit for the hundred-meter dash in the Olympics now stands at a little under ten seconds. From the standpoint that human potential is limitless, this record could conceivably be whittled down to eight seconds, seven seconds, or even less. Modern man is comparatively taller than his ancestors. If human height continues to increase gradually, in the far distant future some people could reach a height of three or even five meters. Personally, however, I doubt that these things will happen because I do not think they are included in our genetic information.

This may make some people wonder, "I understand that I cannot do anything unless it is written in my genes. But shouldn't I be able to run a hundred meters in ten seconds? That must be written in my genes, too." We cannot conclusively say that the reason most of us cannot run as fast as Carl Lewis is because we lack the ability. It may just be lying dormant because the relevant genes are switched off. Chased by a lion or panther, any one of us might run a hundred meters in ten seconds in response to the crisis. But like all living creatures, human beings cannot go beyond the bounds of what is written in their genes.

In the Chinese tale, "Journey to the West," the character Songoku, a monkey, is challenged by the Buddha to escape from the palm of his hand. He travels great distances, marking five pillars in different lands to prove where he has been only to find that this was an illusion. He has merely marked the five fingers on the Buddha's hand. Songoku exhibited fantastic powers, but these powers still did not transcend the power of the Buddha. Similarly, we may exhibit fantastic new abilities, but they do not transcend what is already in our genes, waiting to be discovered. Our genes can even make possible those things we think are impossible.

Miracles do happen. The majority of miracles involve the realization of something humans assume to be impossible. Genetically speaking, however, miracles are part of the program. We are all born with the potential to become living miracles.

Talent Can Bloom at Any Age

There are three factors involved in activating genes: the genes themselves, the environment, and the mind. I think that of these three, the genes are perhaps the most misunderstood. Many people believe that inherited characteristics never change. If they are poor at science or math, they immediately blame it on their parents' lack of ability. Likewise, their parents give up any expectations for their children, believing that nothing can be done. It is true that intelligence and athletic ability are related to genes. But this does not mean that the individual is devoid of these qualities altogether. They are there but have not yet been turned on. Otherwise, how could we explain the existence of a genius? A genius is someone whose genes, inherited from previous generations, are suddenly activated by something. The fact that the children of a genius are often quite ordinary may be because the genetic switch turns on and off from one generation to another.

It is possible that our genes contain not only the memories and abilities passed down from one generation to the next but also those from the entire evolutionary process that spans several billion years. That the human embryo during gestation repeats the process of evolution within the womb suggests that this information is contained within the genes of the first cell. The potential of the entire human race is contained within the genes of the individual. This is why parents who excel should not be disappointed in a child who does not. A mediocre performance simply means that the child's genes are not turned on—yet. You can never tell when something will stimulate their talents.

Genes do not age. With a few exceptions, the genes you have as a teenager are still the same when you are in your eighties. If genes aged, you could not pass genetic information on to your descendants. Therefore, we can assume that genes do not age, at least not fundamentally. If you lead an ordinary life, your genes will change very little. Although they can change in response to unusual external factors such as radiation or harmful drugs such as thalidomide, for the most part they remain stable. It is never too late to develop your potential.

I have heard people blame physical weakness or other perceived failings in their children on the fact that the children were born when the parents were older. But as genes do not age, children born to young parents will not automatically be superior to children born to parents in their fifties. The famous Japanese author Natsume Soseki was born when his parents were so advanced in age that he was called a "shame child." Far from being disadvantaged in any way, he left behind a great legacy. We have the capacity to bloom at any time in our lives, regardless of how old we are. Anything is possible as long as we have the passionate desire and energy to do it. The only obstacle to its achievement is the thought, "I can't do it."

It is never too *early* to start developing potential either, which is why prenatal education is so important. By prenatal education, I mean that the pregnant mother consciously chooses to listen to good music, read good books, see good art, and talk lovingly to the unborn child to educate it. It also consists of avoiding things that inspire negative emotions, because these are considered harmful to the fetus.

We should also remember that each person's genes are unique. A father may have been good at math, but that does not automatically mean his children will excel at the same subject. There are countless examples of artists born into families that have shown no previous signs of artistic ability.

Children born to parents who both have high IQs do not automatically have greater intelligence. In fact, it is far more common for such children to have lower IQs, while children born to parents with low intelligence are more likely to have higher IQs. We do not know why, but genes appear to move toward the mean value. If human beings were programmed with the potential for limitless increase in ability, then they would also carry the potential for the opposite, limitless decrease in ability. As this would jeopardize the survival of the human race, it seems that nature automatically makes some form of adjustment to prevent it. The goal of nature is diversity. It does not matter whether people with high IQ intermarry, nor is it more or less advantageous for people with lower IQ to intermarry. Regardless of the combination, the potential is still the same. Anyone can develop the wonderful talents that lie dormant inside. All they have to do is learn to activate their genes.

III

Your Attitude and Environment Can Change Your Genes

A New Environment Can Act as a Catalyst

Let me begin this chapter by relating how a change in environment activated my own genes. More than thirty years ago, I came to the United States to work as a research assistant at a university. I was fresh out of graduate school and armed with a recommendation from Hisateru Mitsuda, one of my professors. It was that decade in America which made me into a real scientist.

Who knows what I would have become if I had remained in Japan? I do not think that I would have succeeded in the field of science. As a student, I spent more time playing around than attending classes. All my energy and enthusiasm were reserved for joint activities with students from a women's university such as hiking expeditions, parties, and reading circles, and I had distanced myself from friends who were only interested in studying. Needless to say, my grades left much to be desired.

Years later when my research work began appearing in the media, my former classmates were stunned that I was the same Kazuo Murakami they once knew. At class reunions, they always claim that I am the one who has changed the most.

The Japanese university system was part of my problem. Universities were like ivory towers, indifferent to what went on in the world outside. Their bold assertion that they were too busy "investigating truth" seemed impressive, but frankly it was an excuse for doing nothing. At the university, it was possible to do just that. Some professors boasted that their research would only be properly recognized after a century had passed. How could they expect anyone to recognize work like that?

Japanese universities also adhered to a strict hierarchy. Students would never have dared to dream of someday surpassing their professors in rank. These same universities are now coming under fire for their blind obedience to convention, peace-at-any-price philosophy, and bureaucratic approach aimed solely at self-preservation. These were, however, inherent characteristics when I was a student.*

At that time, professors were ensconced at the summit of the university hierarchy followed by assistant professors, lecturers, research assistants, and finally students. Even if you had the capacity, it was—and still is—difficult to rise to the top. Many young, aspiring research assistants find this system not only unpleasant but so void of future prospects that they move to other countries and cause a "brain drain" for Japan.

As for me, I had already resigned myself to becoming a research assistant. I knew that it would be next to impossible

---

* Japan has taken bold steps to address these flaws in its academic system. The Tsukuba Advanced Research Alliance (TARA), established in July 1994, promotes advanced, interdisciplinary research through collaboration among government, industry, and academia—previously distinctly separate. Scientists are recruited from all over the world, not just Japan. Research projects at TARA are reevaluated after a specific period of time by objective third parties. Many universities have adopted TARA's measures, and in addition, they are abandoning the system under which everyone receives the same salary regardless of whether they work hard or just sleep in the lab. Grant recipients are increasingly being selected on the basis of their performance. As a result, universities are now attracting and retaining more students.

to rise to the position of professor. After all, I was not the type of student to inspire high expectations from anyone. But I believed that I would be content to remain in the lower ranks for the rest of my life. Fortunately, I was given the opportunity to go to the United States. Although America is a highly competitive society compared to Japan, it suited me perfectly, and I found myself transformed into an ambitious man.

As we've seen in the enzyme-producing gene that was activated when *E. coli* bacteria were given nothing to eat but lactose, formerly dormant genes can be sparked to action when exposed to a new environment. The genes set to work immediately as if they have just been waiting for this chance. I believe this same phenomenon applies to humans. A new stimulus in a new environment can cause sudden transformation. The Japanese often say, "Change your attitude and apply yourself." This change in mind-set can awaken genes you never even knew you had.

In my case, a new environment in the West challenged my notions of what it was to be a researcher and professor. I was surprised to see how hard the professors applied themselves. They worked and studied from morning until night on their own initiative. They went home for supper, but it was not unusual for them to return to work later that night. Just like the boss of a small company, if a professor does not demonstrate a willingness to work or strive to reach the top, his students will lose faith and abandon him.

American professors constantly stop by to ask research staff, "What's new?" With scientific research, you should count yourself lucky if you come up with something new even once a year. University professors are well aware of this fact. But they still make the rounds every day, almost to the point of obsession. Sometimes a professor will ask this question at noon and then come back in the evening to demand, "What's new tonight?" A development in such a short space of time is highly unlikely, but the professors in my new environment were fanatical about keeping abreast of the latest information.

I was awed by their vitality and enthusiasm for research. I soon realized, however, that this dedication is necessary in the competitive field of scientific research. Even the position of a Nobel Prize laureate is not secure. The award offers prestige for only a few years. If you remain idle after receiving a Nobel Prize, you will be forced to quit. Research grant screening committees, members of which are often young professors or assistant professors, will bluntly inform you that you must give up your research. Like in the world of sumo wrestling, as long as you are winning, you will continue to rise in rank, but even a *yokozuna* who commands the place of honor at the top of the hierarchy will be forced to retire when he hits a losing streak. Anyone who does not produce good work after a note-worthy award like the Nobel Prize is relegated to the past, which shows just how intense the competition is.

If the system is hard on professors, it is naturally even worse for the lower ranks such as research assistants. As a research assistant, if you do not achieve anything noteworthy within three years, you have no right to complain when you are fired. Many people around me lost their jobs while I was there. Someone might be a professor one day only to switch jobs and become a taxi driver the next.

This approach, which is representative of a competitive society, is inconceivable in a Japanese university. If a Japanese Nobel Prize laureate expressed interest in a particular research project, no one would think of saying no. Nor would a pro-fessor be fired for failing to produce any remarkable research. The high esteem awarded to Nobel Prize laureates in Japan may be partly due to the fewness of their numbers. There are only eight compared to two hundred American Nobel laureates. But I am convinced that the difference in treatment also arises from fundamental differences in our environments. In Japanese universities, a professor rules over his students like a feudal lord, and young research assistants who wish to be promoted up the ranks must pledge allegiance to him. In contrast, if a professor in America appears weak and unreliable, his students, far from being loyal, will drop him quickly for fear that they will never get ahead. The two systems are obviously very different.

Of course, there are some drawbacks to a highly competitive system. But for me, steeped as I was in the lukewarm Japanese academic world, everything in America seemed refreshingly new and invigorating, making me feel that the work was worth doing.

Having the opportunity to work alongside Nobel Prize laureates was also very stimulating. In Japan, they are not only scarce but also placed in a class apart. In the United States, they are numerous and accessible, which means that students can envision themselves reaching that level someday. In fact, everyone's goal is to win the Nobel Prize, whereas most Japanese students could not even conceive of doing that. Working alongside Nobel Prize recipients makes you realize that although they certainly have many admirable traits, they are still human, just like you. That opens your eyes to the possibilities; you start to think that you can do it, too. I found this environment, which makes people acutely aware of potential, very attractive.

Growth Occurs through Movement

I have learned from experience that when you reach a dead end, it pays to be daring and to change your environment. For human beings, growth is achieved through movement. A drastic change in environment and exposure to new things can create the perfect opportunity for activating dormant cells. You have probably heard of students who become responsible once they start dorm life despite the fact that they never did any chores or studied when they lived at home. Of course, sometimes the opposite is true, but in general people tend to grow and move forward rather than backward.

Many American students do their undergraduate studies at one university, their master's degree at another, and their doctorate at yet another. This exposes them to many different teachers. Although continuity may be a problem, they have the advantage of movement. In addition, once every seven years, professors in the United States take a sabbatical. They are awarded the privilege of leaving the university entirely and doing whatever they like. This experience is very meaningful and a great opportunity to become refreshed. The majority of professors spend the year in another country, being exposed to a completely different culture. Most Americans go to Europe. The point is that these universities provide an opportunity for professors to get away from the workplace and discover new ideas and research topics.

For Susumu Tonegawa, this type of movement led to the Nobel Prize for Physiology or Medicine. Tonegawa first moved from Japan to the United States to do graduate studies in molecular biology. It was there that he began to truly excel in his field. Subsequently, he spent several years in Europe, where he was involved in groundbreaking research and then returned to the United States to launch a new research project, going on to receive the Nobel Prize in recognition of his achievements.

Without such opportunities, it is difficult to be inspired with new ideas. I recommend that you step out of your normal routine from time to time to see what other places and people have to offer. If you stay in the same place and do the same job without changing your environment or the people with whom you interact, everything else will remain static too, including your point of view. If you remain in the same environment without ever feeling out of place, you will never know life beyond its confines. Shake up your habits regularly to become refreshed and invigorated—mentally and physically.

A change in environment can make you see new things and become the start of a new life. My encounter with the enzyme renin, which was to become my life's work, was the result of such a change. At the time, my position on the faculty of the Vanderbilt University Medical Center in Nashville, Tennessee, was in jeopardy. I had not produced any remarkable research results, and my lectures received poor ratings from students because of my broken English. The economy of the United States, which was just emerging from the disastrous Vietnam War, was in recession, and consequently the performance of foreign professors like myself was judged more harshly than that of our American counterparts.

Dr. Stanley Cohen, a rather eccentric professor, happened to work near my lab. A decade later he was awarded the Nobel Prize, but when I first met him I never dreamed that he would become a world-renowned scientist. In contrast to most Nobel Prize winners whose labs are bustling with activity and attract young researchers, Cohen had only two research assistants and his laboratory was the smallest and the shabbiest in the entire medical center. He certainly did not look like Nobel Prize material. Furthermore, in that modest setting, he was conducting research on growth hormones in mice. Eschewing the latest equipment, he relied instead on the most primitive, outdated research methods, injecting mice with specific substances and observing the results. Although he boasted that he had succeeded in extracting and purifying the growth hormone from salivary glands, he also tended to complain a lot, and at the time, I thought him an uninspiring old man.

One day, he rushed into my lab and exclaimed, "I think I might have made a great discovery. This hormone not only controls growth but is also related to blood pressure. Why don't you help me with my research?" As I had not produced any remarkable research myself, I did not feel I was in a position to refuse him, and so I spent the next year studying whether this growth hormone and the hormone that raised blood pressure were the same. What we discovered after one year of research was that Cohen had made a mistake. Despite his claims that the extract was a pure product, it actually contained a small trace of another substance—the enzyme renin, which is known to be a prime factor in hypertension.

Thanks to this research, I began studying this enzyme and later became the first to decipher the genetic code of human renin. If I had not met and assisted Cohen and if he had not made that mistake, my life would have been very different. Perhaps I was unconsciously seeking to change my research environment due to anxiety about my future. I say "unconsciously" because if I had consciously decided to change my research topic, I would certainly have chosen something different. I later learned that most scientists had steered clear of research aimed at identifying the true nature of renin because of the risks involved.

All previous efforts by well-known scientists to purify renin, which were conducted over several decades, had failed, and consequently the enzyme had a bad reputation among scientists. Researching the subject was regarded as taboo. As I certainly could not expect to achieve results where many great scientists had already tried and failed, given a choice I would have selected a topic that offered more promising results.

Once I began, several people advised me against it, a subject I will touch upon later. It is clear, however, that by assisting Cohen I changed my research environment and the result was a new life. If I had not met him, I would either have been fired or would have returned dejectedly to Japan of my own accord with my tail between my legs. And if I had returned to Japan at that time, I most certainly would have given up research altogether and found some other type of work.

Information Can Change Your Life

In addition to a change in environment, information is another factor that can transform your life. To proclaim that information is important may seem passé in today's information society, but I am talking about information obtained directly through personal communication, a source that is often overlooked.

Information in the world of science consists of two kinds: official information available from established, recognized sources and unofficial information obtained from personal sources. In research situations, the latter is often crucial. It is simple to obtain. You just have to meet with a broad spectrum of people outside the workplace. The most common form of information gathering is wining and dining. Over a glass of wine, you might start out by sharing the type of research you are currently involved in. In response, the other person may share what they or others are doing. This type of exchange is important not just in the field of research but whatever your career aspirations and interests.

Information is crucial to success in scientific research. In my experience, the more capable the scientist, the more effort he or she will invest in being the first to obtain reliable unpublished information. A Japanese professor with whom I worked excelled in this area. He had been living in the United States for thirty years, and his research results were impressive. I noticed that he never ate when attending gatherings of scholars and scientists. When I asked him why, he said, "How can I possibly eat? There might be someone here that I will never have the opportunity to meet again in my life." Meeting as many people as possible was much more important than the food.

Once I attended a seminar where all the participants stayed at the same hotel for several days. About one hundred students were in attendance. Although professors were allotted private rooms, this particular professor chose to share a room with several graduate students because it gave him the chance to hear young people's views and to strike up friendships. He was that eager to gather information. Sharing the same room for a week could be the start of important friendships, and extended personal networks established in this way can be useful for gathering information. A single piece of information, he argued, could change one's entire life. He may be right.

Different ways of networking and gathering information abound. Some people find weekly church, synagogue, or temple services a regular, opportune time to exchange information and gather news. Whatever your interests and passions, being active in a like-minded community or professional organization gives you a chance to stimulate your genes and awaken your potential. Exchanging information through personal relationships can change your life. Don't let opportunities pass you by.

The Value of Cooperation

Another aspect of an environment that helps turn on beneficial genes is one in which hard work is rewarded. Knowing that you will get back what you put into something motivates people to work harder.

Competition occurs in every part of human society, and in my experience scientific research is a constant struggle for fame. For scientists, the chance to see their name "in lights" is when they have a research paper published. The number of papers and the medium in which they are published, as well as the response, determine a scientist's value. Although the names of every person involved in the research are published with the paper, the top name has maximum value because the achievements presented are all attributed to that person. Consequently, conflict often erupts over whose name should come first.

Under such a system, some people's achievements can go unrecognized despite diligent effort simply because they rank lower on the totem pole. If this happens regularly, they will become discouraged, and an enthusiastic and capable person may even decide to quit. Either way, the laboratory will cease producing good research.

This is the conventional way of doing things, but I do not follow it in my lab. Instead, in my lab the person who has worked the hardest on the research comes first on the list, regardless of past experience, achievements to date, or rank. The last name is given to the leader of the research group.

Group leaders are usually assistant professors or lecturers. If the group leader's name has appeared at the end of the list for four or five consecutive years, his or her ability as a leader will be recognized with a promotion. In other words, in our case the results reported in any one paper are the achievements of the person who has worked the hardest and the group leader who will be promoted after four or five years. In this system, everyone knows that his or her efforts will be rewarded.

Perhaps you are wondering whether there is any merit in it for the professor, who is essentially the boss. If my lab consistently produces excellent results and gifted researchers under this system, our lab's reputation will increase. As professor, these will be considered my achievements. Under this system, everyone wins.

Stories of people in power taking credit for the work of their subordinates are common in any field. This approach stems from the premise that the underdog can do the same thing on reaching the top. But in the end, everyone loses. Genetically speaking, it's as if the leader is switching off the good genes of the lower-ranked members, one by one, until finally the entire group loses its motivation—and it is the leader who must bear responsibility for weakening the organization.

In your various roles at work, in your family, and in your community, you most likely have a few that require you to be a good leader. It's important to remember that recognition is an essential component of ensuring that the group succeeds in its goals. When achievements and qualities go unvalued, you can almost feel the morale of the group deflate. Rewarding hard work and good deeds and maintaining a spirit of cooperation is one of the best ways to keep any group functioning smoothly. Plus, you just may be benefiting from the activated genes of those around you.

Practicing "Give and Give" Is an Effective Way to Turn On Your Genes

Most people believe that give and take is the basis of all human relationships, and it is true that most successful personal and business relationships are based on this principle. They also see it as the concept underpinning filial duty or social obligation and responsibility. I, on the other hand, have found that "give and give" is closer to the truth. If you want to turn on your genes, an attitude of give and give is much more effective.

Give and take means that when I give something, I will get something in return. But if you think about it, most "returns" are really nothing to get excited about; they are merely a natural outcome, like getting a train ticket when you put money in the vending machine. We receive the greatest returns from the Divine. It is best to approach life with an attitude of "give and give."

The most typical example of give and give is that of a mother and child. A mother gives to her child constantly without expecting anything in return. She is not consciously expecting a reward, yet she does gain contentment and happiness through her actions. Those feelings of joy and inspiration in turn activate her beneficial genes.

Some scholars of Nobel Prize caliber in America share what they know with everyone, whereas others keep it to themselves while skillfully extracting information from others. Both excel at their work, but the latter usually fail to train new resources. People flock to those who practice give and give. They gather, grow and develop, and create a "family" unit. That family becomes a source of strength, much like when ethnic communities and families come together to exchange news.

In contemporary scientific research it is no longer possible for a single genius depending solely on inspiration and hard work to obtain significant results. Joint research is the current trend, with teams of several people, or even several dozen people, working on a single theme. The study of living organisms makes one thing clear: the head is not the most important part of the body. In fact, there is no hierarchy, as every part performs an irreplaceable role. Although there are many ways to manage an organization, I feel that I have found the ideal system through my genetic research, which has shown me the beauty of how each organ functions and, particularly, of how, despite each cell's independence, all the organs and tissues are exquisitely integrated to form a living organism. We could learn much from this example and apply it to how we interact in our lives.

To Tap Your Power, Put Yourself in a Tight Spot

As the previous examples help illustrate, the right environment and attitude can help activate your good genes and allow you to reach your potential. We certainly have enormous potential, but I have found that sometimes in order to tap it we must be driven into a corner. A cornered mouse will attack a cat: it inherently possesses the power to fight back. I personally would rather put myself in a tight spot than be cornered by someone else. I find that the best way to do this is to "pay my own way." In other words, if you want to succeed at your goal, you have to invest in it. For this reason, I frequently advise my graduate students and staff, "Invest your savings in your research for the first three years, even if you have to talk your family into letting you. Within three years, things will start working out." In the end, perseverance always prevails. In almost every case, investing all your money in your research for three years pays off, and if not, it means that either you lack the necessary ability or luck was not in your favor. But in the cases I have seen, it almost always works out, and when it does, the funds will follow. Projects that produce results attract money, and conversely, no results means no funding.

A professor I greatly respect once told me this story about taking out a loan: When he told the bank manager that he intended to use the funds for research, the manager said that he was the first person who had ever come to borrow money for research rather than to build a house or pay for their children's education. This professor had no collateral, but the bank manager loaned him the money anyway on the condition that he take out a life insurance policy.

Lending money to someone without collateral is highly unusual, but the professor's determination seemed to impress the bank manager, and he took the courageous step of suggesting life insurance as collateral. The professor borrowed a large sum of money that amounted to several times my annual income. (This was twenty years ago.) His willingness to take that risk and invest everything in his research, however, paid off and funding soon came. The initial sum that he paid out of pocket was seed money. I learned from his example, plunging deeply into debt at one point. But if you do not sow the seeds, there will be no harvest to reap.

I have seen this kind of investing in yourself pay off for people in many different areas of business as well. An acquaintance of mine once started a restaurant financed solely by his own savings. The restaurant business is tough in general—but even more so for those just starting out. Putting his own money toward his dream had him in a tight spot, which made him even more determined to make his business a success. His risktaking, hard work, and passion paid off, and the restaurant is now a fixture of the community and enjoying long-term prosperity. He credits "paying his own way" as one reason for his success.

"Paying your own way" is a sure way of introducing risk into your life—one that compels you to strive even harder to reach your goals.

Characteristics of People Whose Beneficial Genes Are Turned On

In my experience, people who are successful and produce the results they want have one thing in common. They have a positive outlook on life. One of my former students is a good example. Several years after joining my laboratory at Tsukuba University, he came to me one day and said, "Could you give me a recommendation so that I can transfer to someplace better? If possible, I'd like to work in a lab that has received a Nobel Prize for research." This student had actually failed to pass the entrance exams to Tsukuba on his first attempt, indicating to me that his aspirations exceeded his ability. Although his request seemed a little impertinent, I sent him off to America with the help of a friend of mine who was working under a Nobel Prize laureate.

Although he was enthusiastic about his research, this student had not been particularly outstanding in Japan. Once in America, however, his brilliance began to shine forth. When he returned to Japan, instead of making him do the usual menial jobs, I assigned him a graduate student and let him concentrate on his research. But I told him, "You are a professor for three years. But just three years. If you have not produced results within that time, you're fired." Just as I anticipated, he produced great results while he was still in his thirties and was recruited as a professor by a prestigious Japanese university. This was unprecedented in the Japanese research environment, where you cannot rise to the top without climbing up through the ranks in the proper order, and in your thirties you can only rise to the rank of assistant professor at best.

Some years earlier I announced my intention of producing the first Japanese professor under forty from my lab. I myself became a full professor at age forty-two, and I actively encouraged my students to aim higher. Apparently, at this particular student's wedding I went so far as to inform his parents that I would make him a professor while he was still in his thirties. Although I had completely forgotten, he remembered and, evidently, took me at my word. The brunt of responsibility for success or failure lay squarely on his shoulders, and this fact seems to have inspired him. In my thinking, at that point in time the genes that would make this happen switched on inside him.

He was also helped along by several fortunate coincidences. One was the realization of his dream to work under a Nobel Prize laureate. I just happened to run into an American friend at a seminar and, remembering that he was working for a Nobel Prize laureate, I asked him if he could help. "I have an eager graduate student who wants to work under a Nobel Prize recipient," I told him.

"That's perfect," he replied. "We were just looking for someone. We'd be glad to take him on." Everything fell into place. But if the student had not told me he wanted to change research labs, my American friend and I would have talked about something else. Luck, it seems, was with him.

He was also fortunate in another way. Joining a lab with a Nobel Prize laureate can have disadvantages. Many research laboratories where the director has reached the pinnacle of success and fame have, along with their director, passed their prime and therefore do not always provide the best research environment. But the lab he joined was producing outstanding results and was headed for a second peak.

He was fortunate when he returned to Japan, too. As a rule, you cannot bring home research achievements from overseas. This was true in his case as well, but he was able to change the subject of his research in such a way that he could continue using the same knowledge and materials. Luckily the nature of his research topic permitted this.

Finally, he was blessed with a certain type of personality. In addition to having a positive outlook, he was able to devote himself solely to the work at hand without worrying about the future. In my experience, this type of character is common in successful people and likewise is a trait of people whose genes are switched on.

The Genes—and Abilities— of Every Individual Are Unique

To achieve success in whatever you aim to do, it's important that the environment and system you work within honors your uniqueness. You may have heard before that every person is unique, but this statement is scientifically true as well. No two sets of genes, or "genomes," are identical. Those areas of our genetic makeup that are not crucial vary slightly from one person to the next. Think of the face. Although every face shares the same basic features, including two eyes, a nose, and a mouth, their size and shape as well as position will differ so that no two people are ever exactly identical. The same is true for genes. Our genomes share common features, but no two people have exactly the same genomes. The differences are manifested not just in a person's looks or physique but also in their character and abilities. When I insist that everyone is endowed with amazing capacities, this is not just to make people feel better. It is literally the truth.

The current education systems in most advanced countries, however, go against the diverse nature of our genes. The focus of the systems is on standardized tests and university entrance examinations. Students are evaluated by fixed standards that measure their ability to memorize and reproduce a specific body of knowledge. Yet each individual is endowed with a unique and diverse set of genes, and the timing and methods by which those genes are activated differ. Therefore, a standardized system cannot possibly cultivate the capacities of every student.

We should, of course, teach knowledge, but systems that are based solely on how much a student can memorize evaluate only a limited section of the abilities latent within us.

The ability to spew out a previously memorized answer is hardly going to contribute to the progress or development of the world. Innovative ideas start from the point where there are no answers, yet students who excel under such systems appear to be at a loss when it comes to exploring the unknown. Memorization is an important ability, but it is not always compatible with searching for new discoveries or creating something new.

It's interesting to note that many Nobel Prize laureates were not particularly outstanding students, at least not in terms of academic performance. When I met Kenichi Fukui, who was awarded the Nobel Prize in Chemistry in 1981, he told me that he had recently failed to solve a chemistry problem from the Japanese university entrance exams even though it was in his field of expertise. "Education today seems to be just memorization, cramming words into your head, and then spitting them out on paper," he remarked. "A person's ability or worth shouldn't be judged on that alone."

My mentor, Ko Hirasawa, was a good friend of Hideki Yukawa, winner of the Nobel Prize in Physics in 1949, making him Japan's first Nobel Prize laureate. Once Hirasawa complained to Yukawa, "My mind works much more slowly than yours. I'm having so much trouble." But Yukawa responded, "You know, I'm having even more trouble with that than you." When Hirasawa confided that he had suffered from a terrible inferiority complex all through junior and senior high school, Yukawa responded, "Me, too!" They were not being modest—just honest.

Both of these brilliant men had poor self-esteem. When I heard this story long ago, it gave me hope that perhaps I, too, could become a professor because I, too, doubted my intelligence. When I was studying for the university entrance exams, my marks were at the cutoff level and I was sure that I had barely scraped through the exams for Kyoto University. I remember being quite relieved to find that there were many other students like me once I got in. Hirasawa and Yukawa were not stupid, but neither of them were standout students by advanced countries' educational standards.

Retaining current education systems around the world with their emphasis on rote memorization and unthinking obedience to rules is unwise, as the value of this type of "intelligence" is rapidly dropping. In the world of business, companies are already announcing that they no longer need employees who passively do what they are told and never think for themselves. This is one indication that society as a whole is moving away from percentile-focused education. Now is the time to invest in the creation of valuable human resources, technology, and intellectual property that will benefit the entire human race. These represent the highest contribution to the international community. Genetically, we are entering an age in which each individual must develop and use their inherent abilities.

People cherish many hopes, but few realize those dreams. If we could switch on our genes, with their three billion pieces of information, anything should be possible. Until recently, we believed that there was nothing we could do to tap into our unused portion. Now that scientists have begun to examine the human mind more deeply, we are beginning to realize that we can tap into this unused potential. For a full and happy life, we must use our minds to activate our genes. Exposure to new things, new information, and new environments are perfect opportunities to stimulate genes that are switched off. This belief is based on all the relevant scientific discoveries to date as well as on my own experience. That is why I recommend living with your genes switched on.

IV

Life Lessons from the Lab

"Night Science" Leads to Great Discoveries

Behind great discoveries or inventions, you'll often find interesting inside stories. Take cell fusion, for example. Current technology enables us to fuse human cells with fungi, but this possibility was discovered purely by accident. A student was conducting an experiment, but it failed every time even though he followed his professor's instructions to the letter. In frustration, he threw in a substance that seemed totally unrelated to the instructions. Fusion took place and led to the new discovery. Even unrelated activities like the custom of exchanging news at family get-togethers can lead to great discoveries.

I call this behind-the-scenes aspect "night science" as opposed to "day science," which consists of lectures, examining objects under the microscope, or presenting research findings at various meetings. Day science is rational and objective with a clear and orderly logic. Night science, on the other hand, derives important clues from intuition, inspiration, and unusual experiences—in other words, from human faculties and events that are not usually associated with scientists. You might say that day science is the tangible results of research while night science is part of the process by which those results are realized. The majority of great scientific discoveries and inventions actually begin with night science. If day science represents left-brain thinking, then night science represents right-brain or, in my terminology, genetic thinking. In this chapter, I would like to share some of the insights I have gained through my own experiences as a scientist concerning intuition, persistence, and the activation of dormant genes.

First, surprisingly, it is important not to know too much when embarking on new research. Knowledge and information are important tools, but when scientists rely exclusively on day science, they can become disadvantaged. It can cause them to take a cautious approach to innovation. Scientists with extensive knowledge are almost always the first to oppose getting involved in new research. The more knowledgeable a person is, the more likely he or she is to be dubious of a new research venture. In contrast, inexperienced people are more likely to launch into something new without hesitation. "Ignorance is bliss" because it allows them to leap right in. This fearlessness often results in great achievements. Buckminster Fuller, one of the key innovators of the twentieth century, put it another way: He advised being a generalist rather than a specialist.

I once asked Masaru Ibuka, a founder of Sony Corporation, to share the secret behind his success in creating a global enterprise. "In retrospect," he told me, "I think that I was lucky not to be an expert." Sony developed Japan's first tape recorder and also introduced transistor technology to Japan. "If I had fully understood tape recorders or transistors at the time," Ibuka remarked, "I would have been far too intimidated to attempt such a thing. When I learned more about them later, I was aghast at my own foolhardiness." I know exactly what he means.

As I mentioned in the previous chapter, my involvement in the study of renin, which was to become my life's work, began with a misinterpretation of data. When I first started research, many of my colleagues advised me to quit. To study renin, a scientist needs pure samples. Although we know that renin is found in the kidneys, the amount is minuscule and also highly unstable. The combination of these two factors amounts to the worst possible conditions for research.

Many scientists had studied renin before me, but no one had succeeded in purifying it. Consequently, researchers in the medical field were actively discouraged from choosing it as a research subject. As my own background was in agricultural chemistry, however, I had never heard of this notorious enzyme, and I plunged in without any hesitation. If I had belonged to the medical department instead of the agricultural department and had known how many people had tried and failed before me, I would never have chosen this field. I have been studying renin ever since, and under Tadashi Inagami at Vanderbilt University, I even succeeded in purifying and manufacturing it. Like Sony's Ibuka, I was lucky not to be an expert, or I would not have attempted this area of science.

I have had many similar experiences of being better off with less knowledge rather than too much. When our research on renin seemed to hit a dead end, for example, we

introduced genetic engineering despite our complete ignorance of the subject. Learning that new technology made it
possible to use *E. coli* bacteria to manufacture human hormones, I thought, "Perfect! Let's use them to make renin."
This was my first exposure to genetic engineering, and once
again, it was probably fortunate that I knew nothing about it.
As a result, we won the race to crack the genetic code for
human renin.

When I decided to introduce genetic-engineering technology into our research, I found that the students with the
highest grades were the most pessimistic. They nervously
questioned the wisdom of becoming involved in a field that
we knew nothing about. Of course, I had no idea whether my
theory would work or not, but I believed it was worth trying
precisely because this was a highly advanced form of technology. The students who supported the idea all shared an avid
curiosity. Their response was, "Sounds interesting. Let's try it."
As long as the subject captures their interest, this kind of student does not give up even if the going gets tough, and consequently, they usually get results.

Why does excess knowledge sometimes work against us?
It is not that information itself is inherently bad; rather,

knowing more than others can delude us into believing our judgment to be superior. Overdependence on knowledge dulls our intuition and can make us look too far ahead. When an endeavor does not proceed smoothly, excessive knowledge can cause us to jump to conclusions; the conclusion reached in such a situation is likely to be pessimistic; and we assume the project is doomed to failure when there is still a prospect for success.

Leo Ezaki, president of Tsukuba University and recipient of the Nobel Prize in Physiology or Medicine in 1973, has several dos and don'ts for becoming a Nobel Prize winner: (1) don't let yourself be trapped by convention; (2) don't hoard knowledge; and (3) get rid of unnecessary information to make room for new knowledge. In a world that requires originality, you cannot stand out if you rely excessively on old knowledge or information. My advice to people who know a great deal is to set aside that knowledge and shut out past experience, at least temporarily.

Failure Isn't an Option When You Have Persistence

When I returned to Japan in the 1970s after completing my work on renin in the United States, I decided to start the same research from scratch at the recently established Tsukuba University. At first, I considered switching to a different subject, but I could not give up renin with its potential for treating hypertension. To study it, however, I needed materials. Around this time, I learned there was a possibility that renin occurs in the brain. Opinion in the scientific world concerning this subject had been split down the middle for twenty years and the majority of scientists favored the hypothesis that it is not found in the brain. On the basis of several pieces of circumstantial evidence, however, my colleagues and I were convinced that renin *is* found in the brain. I decided to obtain an extract of renin from the brain as proof.

The brain contains the pituitary gland, a small sack filled with hormones. Assuming that these glands should contain a large amount, I decided to obtain some of these glands from the brains of cows or pigs. The problem was that I needed a very large quantity. I needed at least one milligram of renin as research material, and calculating backwards from this figure, I estimated that we would need somewhere between thirty and forty thousand brains to obtain it—an overwhelming number! How could we possibly obtain that many pituitary glands?

First, I contacted pig farms near Tsukuba University, but they did not have anywhere near the required number. Next, deciding that Japan's most densely populated city, Tokyo, must have enough, I visited the cattle yards daily and begged them to help until finally they arranged to give us the pituitary glands from slaughtered cattle. Students from our lab traveled to Tokyo several times a month to pick them up, and our project was underway.

A bovine pituitary gland is about the size of the tip of your thumb and is covered by a tough membrane like that of a chestnut, which makes it extremely difficult to peel. "If we can just peel these things," I urged my students, "our research will take the world by storm." In reality, however, there was no way of guessing what the outcome would be. That is the nature of research—you do not know until you try. There is always a possibility but never any guarantee. This is only true, however, in the world of "day science." In the world of "night science," the leader must have unswerving faith in the desired outcome.

Stories exist of people who suffer for many years from an illness such as rheumatism and then are told that a certain remedy, such as a hot spring, will cure them. Convinced that it is true, they find that after bathing in the waters their pain disappears for good. I believe that the change in their thinking switches on dormant, beneficial genes. While the hot spring may have had curative properties, certainly their conviction played a role in curing the illness. In the same way, when a leader decides that a goal is possible, the people around him will believe it, too. But he or she must believe it with all his heart. Many failures occur in life, but every one of them begins from the moment we start thinking that we have failed. Conversely, as long as we refuse to give up and believe that we still have a chance, we have not failed no matter how badly things seem to be going.

As we worked together peeling pituitary glands, we gradually got into the swing of it and began to have fun, chatting as we worked. Encouraged, my little pep talks began to escalate in scale: "This may lead to the development of a remedy for hypertension." "We may be rewarded with a patent worth several billion yen."

Interestingly, when people are enthusiastically involved in something, other people want to join the action. Doctors, graduate students, undergraduates, and in the end even people just passing by came in to help. We peeled all 35,000 pituitary glands, each weighing about 1.5 grams, for a total of about 50 kilograms. After freeze-drying them to make a powder that resembled instant coffee, we succeeded in extracting the renin as anticipated.

Unfortunately, after all that work, the result was only 0.5 milligrams of renin, only half the amount we expected. It was so small that we could not even see it with the naked eye. But at least we had succeeded in purifying renin from the brain.

I immediately announced this finding at the convention of the International Society of Hypertension in Heidelberg in 1979—a selective and prestigious meeting. When I finished my presentation, the room was filled with thunderous applause for the fact that we had put an end to twenty years of international debate concerning the presence of renin in the brain.

I learned a precious lesson from this experience: Successful research depends not on one's scholastic level but rather on being an "early riser." I mean this both literally and in the sense of getting a jump on the competition. When we were peeling pituitary glands, I suggested to my students that we get an earlier start in the mornings, and they all complied. Tsukuba University was still a new and virtually unknown university with a history of less than ten years. I kept telling my research staff that it's like a ballgame: "No one in this university has made a home run yet, but if we keep getting hits, we can still make points. And if you can't make a hit, at least get to first base by walking or by running on the last strike. Let's at least get to first base."

Scientists are always competing against invisible rivals. Because we are all thinking the same things and using similar techniques, the other side will occasionally fumble or walk the batter. You just have to wait for those opportunities. It is the same in other professions as well, be it retail, entertainment, stock exchange, or any number of businesses with a healthy dose of competition. The key to that is to keep on working. Persistence leads to power. As long as you keep on trying, you have a chance. This is the attitude of a winner.

It was thanks to the hard work of everyone on our research team that we finally succeeded in extracting renin. At the reception after my presentation, scientists from around the world came up to congratulate me. Many of them said, "You are lucky that Japan is such an economic giant." I was puzzled by this until someone asked me, "So how much did it cost you to import all those pituitary glands from the States?" Then it dawned on me. They thought I had bought the pituitary glands from America. I proudly told them the truth. "We didn't import them. The slaughterhouse donated them to us.

Everyone—my graduate students and I, other doctors and students, even my wife—helped to peel them." I did not tell them that my wife was the best peeler of all. My nickname thereafter was "Dr. 35,000 Cows."

There Is No Finish Line in Science

Not surprisingly, "Dr. 35,000 Cows" immediately faced another hurdle.

Although to us the renin sample we had so painstakingly extracted seemed a precious treasure, it was not enough. The minuscule 0.5 milligrams that had been greeted with such fanfare may have succeeded in ending an international debate, but it was nowhere near sufficient for our ultimate goal: deciphering renin's genetic code. Moreover, even if it was extracted from brains, it was from cow brains, not human brains, and as the aim of our research was to make a useful contribution to treating hypertension in humans, we were still far from our goal. The ideal solution would have been to collect human renin from human brains, but that was out of the question. Once again I was at a loss.

Having just received international acclaim, this situation was doubly painful. After much agonizing, I decided to adopt a different attitude. "This is the beginning of a new phase," I told myself. "It's a sign that we are about to make a great leap forward." This positive frame of mind allowed me to relax. Soon after, we heard some exciting news: large quantities of human insulin had been successfully produced by *E. coli* bacteria using newly developed technology. We had entered the age of genetic engineering. After consulting with my staff, I decided to introduce genetic engineering into our project even though we knew nothing about it. Our goal was twofold: to produce large quantities of human renin from *E. coli* bacteria and to decipher the enzyme's genetic code.

We were just about to begin decoding the genetic makeup of mouse renin in preparation for this experiment when we received some disheartening news: France's Pasteur Institute, the grand champion of the research world, had already finished decoding mouse renin. Despite this setback, we changed tactics and immediately launched into decoding human renin. The Pasteur Institute, we assumed, could not have gotten that far yet if they had just completed mouse renin.

As renin had already been identified in human kidneys, we decided that it would be easier to extract it from kidneys than brains. To do that, we needed a fresh human kidney with a high renin content—which is not easy to come by. We used whatever we could get, but the results were unsatisfactory. We were running out of time, particularly as I had publicly announced that our research results would be ready for Tsukuba University's tenth anniversary. Then we received another blow. The Pasteur Institute along with Harvard University had not only started on human renin but had already succeeded in decoding 80 percent of it. Although this information was unofficial, it seemed highly probable. Were they going to beat us to the finish again? I flew to France to find out.

In Paris, the Pasteur Institute confirmed the rumor. "You cannot hope to catch up with us at this point. Why don't you try decoding monkey renin instead?" they suggested, smugly confident of their success. The thought of decoding monkey genes after the genetic code for human renin had already been completed seemed such a letdown. Yet they had already decoded 80 percent while we were still looking for material. How could we possibly compete? But often, I have observed, the moment that defeat seems inevitable, miracles begin to happen.

I had flown from Paris to Heidelberg, Germany, to attend a meeting and was drinking a beer in a pub near the university, deeply discouraged, when in walked an acquaintance of mine, Shigetada Nakanishi, a professor at Kyoto University with an international reputation in the field of genetic engineering. He sat down and I poured out the whole story to him.

Nakanishi's response took me by surprise: "They've only decoded 80 percent, right? In that case, you still have a chance. You know, even when people have decoded 99 percent of a gene, very often they get stuck at the last part."

"But we haven't even—"

"If you'd like, I'll get my lab to help."

It was like a gift from heaven. Granted, a conference was being held in the city, but the chance of meeting not only someone I knew but also an expert on genetic engineering such as Nakanishi in a little pub in Germany was one in a million. With him on our side, I felt we still had a fighting chance. We were still at a disadvantage, but I was ready to give it one more shot. Energy and enthusiasm renewed, I cancelled the rest of my trip and returned to Japan immediately.

Fervent Thoughts Are Contagious

Bad news may come in threes, but sometimes good news does, too. There was some of that waiting for me upon my return.

A doctor who had collaborated with us in our lab had informed university hospitals throughout Japan to notify us in the event of surgical removal of a kidney with a large amount of renin. As a result of his efforts, I received a phone call from someone at Tohoku University. "We're removing a kidney tomorrow," he informed me. "Please pick it up immediately." Our staff gathered up some dry ice, and in the middle of the night we drove as fast as we could to the hospital, about two hundred miles away. To our delight, the kidney we obtained contained ten times the normal amount of renin due to the nature of the patient's illness. This was a very lucky break for our team.

Now we were doubly determined to identify the mechanism causing hypertension, not just for our own sakes but also for the sake of the donor. After extracting the renin, we divided our staff between Tsukuba University and the Nakanishi laboratory at Kyoto University and set to work on reading the genetic code of renin. Our rival, the Pasteur Institute, was already nearing the finish line, and here we were just getting started. Graduate students brought sleeping bags to stay over in the lab, and we worked day and night. But we were so excited to be on the brink of a world-shaking discovery that we could not have slept anyway. This last, desperate spurt paid off. When our team finally completed the code, the Pasteur Institute had not yet finished. We were the first to decipher the complete genetic code of human renin—the ultimate goal. It was the height of summer in 1983, just three months before Tsukuba University was to celebrate its tenth anniversary.

A single achievement involves an enormous number of people. In retrospect, this spectacular feat, which won us international acclaim, could not have been achieved without the cooperation of many others: the person at the slaughterhouse who provided all those pituitary glands, the many willing volunteers that helped peel them, the doctor who advertised our need for a fresh kidney, the people at Tohoku University who responded to that plea, and of course, Dr. Nakanishi and his research staff. Although many times I felt discouraged, particularly when faced with a fresh obstacle, it was my positive attitude that pulled me through.

Scientific research and development has a fiercely competitive side, an element of rivalry derived from the egotistical desire for fame and success. Although I acknowledge this aspect, at the same time, I am proud that what I do contributes to humanity. While on the one hand I want to win,

I also maintain an awareness that transcends the immediate outcome, the knowledge that even if I lose the race, there is still meaning in what I do. Those are the times that I feel my beneficial genes are truly activated. And I am confident that as the leader of the group, this feeling is transmitted to my staff and those near to me.

The Japanese often say, "Fervent desires reach heaven," but experience makes me think that perhaps such thoughts are really transmitted to the genes inside our cells rather than to heaven. This is more of a hunch than a scientific truth at this point, but many events in my life lead me to believe this. Take the following story, for example.

Once we had succeeded in decoding human renin, we set ourselves several new goals, one of which was to produce hypertensive mice with human renin genes. As this story is related in full in the next chapter, I will not go into detail here. Suffice it to say that we had problems from the start. No matter what we did, the blood pressure of the mice did not rise. In the midst of this crisis, I was appointed to lead the campaign supporting Leo Ezaki in the election for university president. This kept me away from the laboratory for some time.

Never having been involved in election work before, I was under severe stress, and as a result, my blood pressure started rising. Imagine my surprise when I was told that the blood pressure of our experimental mice had begun rising at the same time. Until then, they had exhibited no signs of hypertension no matter how much we wished that they would, but now it seemed as if their blood pressure was rising in response to mine. I was forced to conclude that it might really be synchronicity. But it gives me reason to believe that fervent thoughts are transmitted to the people—and all living things—around us.

Good Research Results Depend on Intuition

The story of our successful decoding of human renin is also a prime example of the vast rewards of using one's intuition. To achieve good research results, a scientist needs to use his or her intuition. In fact, some people believe that intuition can determine the success or failure of a research project. Intuition plays a part in the success of many endeavors outside of science as well.

We know that it's smart to follow our intuition, but we don't often make the connection to the concrete results in our lives. Take my lab's race against the Pasteur Institute. My gut feelings played a key role in our triumph. As I mentioned earlier, we had not even started decoding the gene whereas the Pasteur Institute was already 80 percent finished. When I fortuitously ran into Shigetada Nakanishi after learning that the Pasteur Institute was almost finished, fate hung in the balance. If I had heard his offer to help and had instead replied, "I appreciate your kind words, but I think we had better pull out now," that would have been the end of the story. Although in retrospect it seems odd, my intuitive reaction was, "God is on our side. We've won!" and I made a choice that from an objective perspective must have appeared very unwise.

When I returned to the lab with my newfound enthusiasm, everyone else caught it too, and their eyes glowed with excitement. Those graduate students who had moved from Tsukuba to Kyoto to work on the project stayed in the lab day and night engrossed in research. We were on an adrenalin rush and finished decoding the gene within three months. The fact that we won the international race to identify the genetic code of human renin against odds of ninety-nine to one was due to the tireless efforts of the graduate students and the flash of intuition that came to me in a pub in

Heidelberg. In addition to illustrating how intuition leads to positive results, it is also a good example of how genes are activated in a crisis.

In the next chapter, I'd like to share with you in more detail the research that followed after we successfully decoded human renin. If you find this information too technical, in chapter 6 we will return to a discussion of the wonder of our genes, how we can live in accordance with nature's laws, and how science and spirituality are intricately linked.

V

The Wonders of the Blueprint of Life

Exciting advances are being made in the field of genetics and gene therapy. Every step we take—no matter how small—brings us closer to comprehending the vast potential contained in our genes and the many ways we can work with them to live fuller, healthier lives. My goal in this chapter is to help illuminate the wonder of our genes—the blueprint of life—and illustrate the ongoing influence of genes in our lives.

Genes Influence Some Factors More Than Others

As I've mentioned, each gene contains a vast amount of information equivalent to thousands of books. As genes are the basic blueprint of every living organism, their content does not change except in unusual circumstances such as mutation. Genetic information is encoded in four chemical bases expressed by the letters A, T, C, and G, the order of which provides the instructions for protein synthesis. A single gene consists of over three billion of these chemical letters. But if even one letter in a sequence is missing, that particular protein cannot be made according to the instructions. For example, an infant will be born without a hand if the gene crucial to its development is damaged.

Similarly, alteration of the gene governing sexual behavior in male fruit flies disrupts the typical courtship pattern. Males may begin pursuing males instead of females, be unable to copulate, remain attached to the female after copulation, or even lose all interest in courting. This clearly demonstrates that genes govern their sexual behavior. In the case of humans, however, sexual behavior is more complex.

We cannot automatically assume that sexual preference in humans is due to genetic factors. In some people it may be genetically rooted, while in others it may derive from environmental influences or factors other than genetic information. One of the genes for a particular sexual tendency that is switched off in the male parent may be activated in the child due to some other stimulus. External stimuli include culture, time factors such as when a person is born, education, and geographical factors such as where they live. At this stage, however, we still do not fully understand how much is governed by genes or what changes are the result of other stimuli.

We do know that genetics significantly influences sexual behavior, which after all directly affects preservation of the species. On the other hand, the environment is believed to play an almost equal role with genes in determining conditions that result in weaker constitutions such as hypertension. Likewise, while genes may determine a person's inherent intelligence, it is reasonable to assume that postnatal factors other than heredity play a major role because development of the individual's abilities is affected by study, experience, and effort. You may have the genetic makeup to be very smart, but the final outcome will vary greatly depending on your childhood experience and how much effort you put into your studies.

As for the role genes play in character and disposition, we are waiting for the results of current genetic research. Although the media have reported the discovery of genes that determine happiness or attract the opposite sex, from a scientific viewpoint these claims should be taken with a grain of salt.

Because they may be true, they should not be rejected outright. But no substantial evidence supports these theories yet. With fruit flies, we can create a controlled environment with fixed external stimuli to study how the genes behave, but as this is impossible for human beings, it is much more difficult to determine the degree of influence.

Although we don't know if there is a gene that determines sex appeal, we do know which gene governs the internal biological clock of living organisms. Our bodies are set to a twenty-four-hour cycle. The tendency to become sleepy at night and wake up in the morning, or conversely, the tendency for nocturnal creatures to become active from sunset, indicates the existence of a gene that controls this cycle. Dubbed the "clock gene," it was first identified in mice in 1977 by a research team at Northwestern University in the United States. Although it had already been identified in bacteria and fruit flies, the discovery of the same gene in mammals is expected to contribute to the development of new remedies for insomnia and jet lag in humans.

We are certain that genes are related to a variety of behaviors. We will understand much more about this in the near future as research continues to make advances. This may make it possible to enhance people's abilities by altering their genes or character. But we should not forget that, in humans, environmental factors also play an important role. Altering a person's genes is meaningless if those genes are not activated.

Genetic Influence on Intelligence

Some outstanding geniuses have graced humankind's history. It is puzzling to many people that the offspring of geniuses are rarely born with the same exceptional qualities. It is far more common for the children of geniuses to be of mediocre ability. Goethe's son, for example, had below-average intelligence as well as a weak constitution. Mozart had many children, but the majority died in infancy, and although one of his two sons became a composer, he was no match for his father. The same trend can be seen with scientific geniuses: only rarely do their offspring or even their siblings exhibit the same talent. This discrepancy, which occurs despite the fact that they all share the same genes, is most likely caused by two factors: environmental influences and the genetic on/off mechanism.

While geniuses exhibit remarkable ability in certain areas, it is often accompanied by eccentricities in other areas. As the children of a genius are exposed firsthand to their parent's idiosyncrasies, it is not surprising that many do not want to grow up to be like that parent. In fact, it seems that both genetic and environmental factors combine to prevent the recurrence of a genius in the family tree.

In the Darwinian theory of evolution, humans, animals, and plants evolved over billions of years. The key concept is survival of the fittest through natural selection. Only those who are strong enough to adapt to a changing environment survive. Essentially, the mechanism involved in evolution is genetic change.

Our genes contain genetic information from our past, including the genes of fish and reptiles. While in the womb, the fetus passes rapidly through the stages of human evolutionary development. In other words, the embryo reenacts the entire sequence of evolution, indicating that the history of evolution is imprinted on our genes. For example, the embryo in the early stages of fetal development takes on the shape of a fish (see figure 5). But humans are never born as fish or reptiles, because at some point during fetal development those genes switch off, or if they do not, the mother's body rejects the fetus, and it is aborted.

Figure 5
Early stages of fetal development

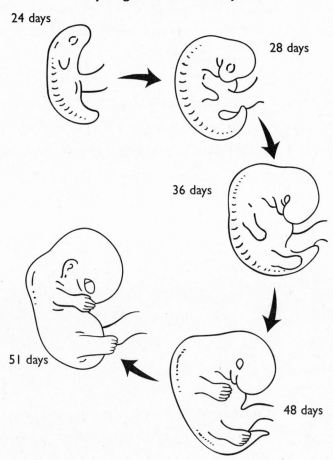

24 days

28 days

36 days

51 days

48 days

Motoo Kimura, a geneticist famous for his theory of neutral evolution developed in response to Darwinian theory, claims that the chance of any living creature being born at all is equivalent to the chance of one person consecutively winning $100 million in the lottery one million times. Some may envy geniuses and prodigies, but if they had to stand in their shoes, they might just find that geniuses experience their own version of pain and suffering. Perhaps geniuses envy those with mediocre ability. Rather than envying each other, however, we should acknowledge the fact that just to be born is a miraculous achievement.

If Key Genetic Information Is Disrupted, Critical Damage Occurs

In chapter 1, I presented the structure of DNA (see figure 2) and described how the four chemical bases, A, T, C, and G, found at the rungs of the helical spiral, are paired: A with T and C with G. These pairs never change, except through mutation. The information encoded by these letters is packed into twenty-three pairs of chromosomes and governs the sequence of amino acids during protein synthesis. Amino acids are the building blocks of protein, and the genes designate the type of protein to be made by specifying the order in which the amino acids are arranged.

Protein is one of the most important components comprising the body. A difference in the order of a single amino acid can change the type of protein. The proteins of vegetables, animals, and humans are all different. Even the proteins comprising muscle tissue vary slightly between, for example, cows and human beings. The difference is determined by the order of the amino acids in the structure of the genes. Therefore, it is the differences in genes that determine one species from another. But we do not know the details of which gene or what part of it marks the dividing line between, for example, a human being and a monkey.

Proteins consist of amino acids arranged in a long, complex sequence, and there are always one or two points in the sequence that play a crucial role in the protein's functioning. These are known as active sites. There are very few active sites compared to the rest of the sequence. Whereas damage to other parts of the sequence seems to make little difference, deletion or mutation of a gene governing an active site will disrupt production of that protein and can result in an obvious abnormality in the organism.

This is similar to the large, seemingly unused portion of our cells and genes. As far as we have been able to discover, only a small percentage of our fifteen billion brain cells are being effectively used, so the number of deactivated genes far exceeds the number of activated genes. But there is meaning in their idleness. Various viruses and bacteria bombard our bodies. If the gene's structure allowed no space to maneuver, the part under attack would be damaged instantly. And the damage would be even worse if this part were vital. In order to prevent this, genes contain empty space despite their small size. This space is certainly not useless. Just compare the amount of damage a missile would do if it hit a densely populated city as compared with a broad desert or forest and you will understand what I mean.

If an abnormality occurs during pregnancy, the baby may be born with a disability or a hereditary illness. In other words, if key information in a gene is defective, it will hinder normal development of the body. Hereditary anemia, for example, occurs because the genes governing the production of hemoglobin are abnormal and so do not produce the necessary protein. Likewise, hemophilia, a blood disorder in which blood does not clot properly, is caused by the absence of a blood-clotting protein. We now know that genetic factors play a much greater role than initially thought in what are usually called "lifestyle diseases" as well, although environmental factors must not be ignored.

Thus, genes are at the root of many illnesses: either a gene has ceased functioning properly or a gene that should not be functioning at all has been activated. The factors that cause these defects can be broadly divided into heredity and the environment. People who are born with a genetic tendency to develop a specific disease may never manifest any symptoms if the environmental factors are favorable. In this case, we can assume that the genes which should have caused the illness have not been activated. For example, if your family has a history of diabetes but you have shown no signs of it, you very well may be carrying the gene, but the environmental factors—possibly including psychological factors—specific to you have kept the gene deactivated.

Renin's Role in Hypertension

I'd like to explain in greater detail the process of our study of renin and the joys and frustrations involved in our particular adventure to help treat hypertension. To give you some background, hypertension is believed to affect one out of every four adults in the United States. Of those who suffer from this condition, 70 percent can now be successfully treated with renin inhibitors and other medications. Scientists first recognized renin as a substance that raises blood pressure at the end of the nineteenth century. Since damage to or malfunction of the kidneys results in high blood pressure, scientists assumed that something in the kidneys must cause hypertension. They made a kidney extract, injected the liquid into a subject's vein, and found that it did indeed raise blood pressure. This substance was named *renin*, which means "kidney." Subsequent research revealed the enzyme/hormone system shown in figure 6. The enzyme renin does not directly raise blood pressure itself but rather stimulates the hormone precursor angiotensinogen, which causes blood pressure to rise by making the hormone angiotensin. This hormone is the most potent hypertensive substance known today. Medicine that inhibits the functioning of this enzyme/hormone system is now widely used to treat hypertension.

The Role of *E. coli* Bacteria in Genetic Engineering

As I mentioned in the previous chapter, my lab won the race to identify the true structure of human renin in large part due

Figure 6
Malfunction of the enzyme/hormone system causes hypertension

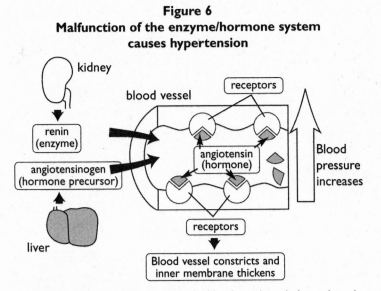

Renin and angiotensinogen react within the blood vessel, producing angiotensin, which bonds with receptors. This causes constriction of the blood vessel, and consequently blood pressure rises.

to *E. coli* bacteria and its valuable role in genetic engineering. Due to outbreaks of some virulent strains, most people view *E. coli* bacteria with fear. Scientists involved in genetic engineering, however, regard this organism with profound respect because it has proved to be a most convenient host for transferring genes. Moreover, it reproduces itself every twenty minutes, which is extremely useful for making copies of transferred genes and for synthesizing proteins based on genetic instructions. *E. coli* has consequently been thoroughly ana-lyzed, making the bacteria ideal research material and the source of many Nobel Prizes. In fact, *E. coli* bacteria are the most frequently used medium in genetic research today. The number of people who have obtained their doctorates from studying these organisms is easily several thousand.

E. coli bacteria contain only 4.6 million pieces of genetic information, compared to three billion for the human genome, another point in its favor as far as research is con-cerned. The complete genetic structure of *E. coli* bacteria was decoded in 1997. This means that we can now identify the difference between the virulent O-157, the 157th strain of *E. coli* bacteria, and ordinary *E. coli* bacteria, making it possi-ble to combat the problems with the most virulent strain at the genetic level.

With the decoding of the renin gene, we were immedi-ately able to identify its basic structure, and on this basis we produced a three-dimensional model in 1985. However, as this model was only an estimate, we wanted to clearly identify its true structure. To do this, we needed a large amount of human renin, and we used *E. coli* bacteria to produce it.

Figure 7 illustrates one way of using *E. coli* bacteria to produce human proteins. This method is used to make such proteins as human insulin, human interferon, and human growth hormones. The technology for exploiting genes in *E. coli* bacteria to produce these proteins was greeted with great excitement. Previously, substances such as interferon, which is believed to be effective in treating cancer, had to be extracted from human subjects, and it took eighteen months to obtain just five milligrams. In contrast, genetic-engineering techniques allow us to produce as much as we want.

We did indeed succeed in making human renin from *E. coli* bacteria. But we encountered our share of difficulties. Although our basic structural model of renin was perfect, the human renin we produced was like a tangle of useless string instead of the beautifully shaped, living, functioning enzyme we had anticipated. Human hormones and proteins manufactured by *E. coli* bacteria are made inside the cells of the bacteria. It is therefore necessary to break the tough cell membrane to extract them. In addition, separating the manufactured substance from the normal *E. coli* proteins is extremely difficult. So we had succeeded in making the correct

Figure 7
Production of human protein from *E. coli* bacteria

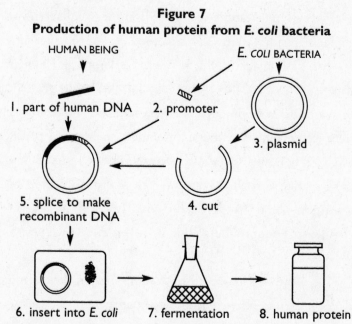

HUMAN BEING

E. COLI BACTERIA

1. part of human DNA 2. promoter

3. plasmid

5. splice to make recombinant DNA

4. cut

6. insert into *E. coli*   7. fermentation   8. human protein

To produce human protein using *E. coli* bacteria, we must splice an *E. coli* bacteria promoter in front of the human structural gene being introduced. The bacterium's RNA synthetase will recognize the promoter, bond with it, and begin transcribing. We use a promoter that includes a regulator gene capable of starting and stopping transcription of the DNA by messenger RNA. Without a regulator we could not control the on/off switch. The promoter's regulating mechanism is initially set in the off position to allow sufficient proliferation. The mechanism is then switched on and the bacteria begin making protein. When we provide lactose or other food to promote *E. coli* bacteria growth, the repressor is released, inducing synthesis. We use plasmids as the carriers of the promoter necessary for protein synthesis and of the DNA fragment necessary for copying DNA. Plasmids are loops of DNA that are not integrated with the pairs of chromosomes that make up the core of our genetic information but rather float freely and replicate independently. As they are easily extracted, we can use them effectively to make desired substances.

amino acid sequence, but it would not form the proper three-dimensional shape of renin. This meant that we could not fulfill our objective of creating a structural model. Realizing that *E. coli* bacteria were not going to work, we decided to try again with three other types of cell: yeast, bacillus subtilis, and a cultured animal cell.

This time we joined forces with Upjohn Company, an international pharmaceutical firm. We decided to work with Upjohn because of the keen interest they evinced, contacting us within a week of our extracting human renin, and because of their insistence on conducting a thorough study beginning from the basic research stage. Their interest stemmed from the fact that we had actually produced human renin. If our techniques could be used to make a large amount, they could crystallize it and analyze its true form for use in developing an effective treatment for hypertension. As a pharmaceutical company, their goal was to make medicine. To do this they needed to identify the true structure of renin as soon as possible. With this knowledge it would be comparatively easy to make a renin inhibitor.

Together we made two hundred milligrams of renin and used it to define the structure of renin (see figure 8).

Research Often Yields Unexpected Results

The production of renin and identification of its structure led to an unexpected development that benefited many people. An enzyme belonging to the same family as renin was subsequently identified as a potentially effective treatment for AIDS. Many companies began working on its development, resulting in a new drug. The number of deaths due to AIDS in the United States dropped in 1997 for the first time since AIDS was discovered, a fact directly related to the intro-

Figure 8
Human renin and inhibitor complex

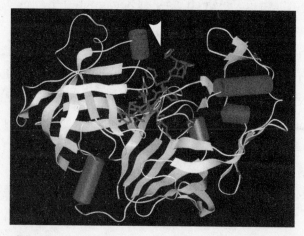

The arrow indicates the inhibitor. The rest is human renin.

duction of this medicine. Our research results also led to development of a hypertension inhibitor, resulting in a 70 percent cure rate for renin-related hypertension. This latter drug has also been introduced in Japan.

The structure of renin was clearly identified between 1990 and 1991, five to six years after we had made our estimated model of human renin. Not only did we achieve our real aim—to learn how to mass-produce human protein using genetic engineering—but the results of our basic research led to the development of treatments for AIDS and hypertension and set the stage for drugs to be designed using computer graphics. So we were very satisfied with the results.

Subsequently, we turned our attention to gene therapy to further explore treatments for hypertension. Gene therapy is a revolutionary technology that represents the future of medicine. In the next section, I'd like to share some of the background and recent advances of this exciting area of genetics.

Cracking the Genetic Code Makes Gene Therapy Possible

Each cell in your body is an independent living organism. A liver cell, for example, must not only function as a liver cell but must also be alive in its own right in order to fulfill that function. How is the human body, which is composed of trillions of cells, formed? It begins with a single fertilized egg, and every cell thereafter is produced by cell division, not acquired from some external source. Even giant sumo wrestlers began as a single fertilized egg, so tiny it was invisible to the naked eye.

The main research methods used in the life sciences are experiments and observation. Dramatic advances in observation technology and experimental methods have made it a fairly simple matter to extract and thoroughly examine organs such as the liver. But when we remove these organs, they are unlikely to function in the same way as when they are inside the body. This is true not only for tissue but for cells as well. If we extract and cultivate a cell in the lab, we can describe what it does but we still do not know if the same thing will occur when the cell is inside the body. We must check whether the individual cell when replaced will function the same way it did in the lab, because although at times it may function identically, other times something totally unexpected happens.

In the developing field of genetic engineering, genetic diagnosis and genetic treatment have generated intense interest. Although the ethical and moral issues remain, the technology for identifying and extracting or deleting a specific gene has already been developed, and genetic manipulation for medical treatment is a natural outcome. A disease could be cured, for example, by deleting the harmful gene causing it. This is known as gene therapy, and the number of disease-causing genes being identified is rapidly increasing. Gene therapy is like artificially controlling the genetic on/off mechanism, and it has the potential to be extremely helpful in the treatment of disease. Animal experiments have already been conducted on introducing a missing gene to overcome functional disabilities, and we are approaching the point where we can manipulate genes at will. At the same time, however, the results can be unpredictable and potentially harmful, as you'll see in the following example. Accordingly, we must be extremely cautious in using this therapy.

In 1988, a research team at Tsukuba University identified the hormone endothelin, which plays a role in constricting blood vessels. This outstanding discovery received international attention because of endothelin's effect on blood pressure even when administered in small amounts. Scientists all over the world rushed to study it. Using the technology that allows us to isolate a specific gene and extract, delete, or replace it, the gene related to endothelin was deleted in mice. As a result, blood pressure stopped rising in the mice. Perceiving potential applications in the treatment of hypertension, scientists produced experimental mice in which this gene was disabled. But soon it became dramatically clear that the gene played a decisive role in the formation of the jaw, because the genetically modified mice were born without lower jawbones. Not being able to breathe, these mice died soon after birth. This goes to show that many unknowns exist in the advancing field of gene therapy.

The process of isolating and disabling a specific gene is known as genetic "knockout." Let me give you a simple explanation of how knockout mice are produced. This technology became possible when scientists discovered how to cultivate embryonic stem cells in the lab instead of in the body. (Embryonic stem cells, like fertilized eggs, can give rise to every type of cell that is found in the adult.) A knockout gene is inserted into a normal embryonic stem cell from the black mouse and then introduced into the embryo of a normal white mouse during the eight-cycle stage (when the cell divides into eight) to produce a hybrid embryo. This embryo is then implanted in the surrogate mother. Knockout mice are produced by breeding the resultant offspring that have been born with the altered gene in their reproductive cells. This method is used to knockout specifically targeted genes.

Gene Therapy Is Risky but Also Revolutionary

To study renin and clarify the mechanism by which hormones raise and lower blood pressure, our research team set out to produce hypertensive mice. Why do we bother producing mice with high blood pressure? Unfortunately, there is no other way to do this; these mice are very useful in developing medicines for the prevention and treatment of hypertension in humans. By experimenting with hypertensive model mice, we can examine how the genes that are involved in the onset of hypertension function and the relationship between genes and such environmental factors as diet.

The Tsukuba hypertensive and hypotensive mice have transferred genes. To produce hypertensive mice, we began by mating normal mice and extracting fertilized eggs from the females. A human renin gene was then inserted into the nucleus of each fertilized egg (see figure 9), and the eggs were implanted in surrogate mothers, which produce litters of about fourteen young. Usually about two of the offspring carry

Figure 9
Inserting gene into fertilized egg

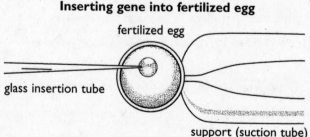

the human renin gene. We found that the human renin genes in the mice promote special kidney cells that produce large amounts of human renin just as they do in the human body. In mice, it was switched on and functioned just as we had expected it to, but their blood pressure remained normal.

Next we made mice that had the counterpart of human renin—the hormone precursor human angiotensinogen. In this case, too, the human gene in the mice was switched on and the livers and other organs produced large quantities of human angiotensinogen. But once again, the mice's blood pressure was normal.

The results demonstrated that the regulator genes in both human renin and human angiotensinogen did indeed function inside mice, just as we had expected they would, a success we owed to thorough research on regulator genes at the cell level. However, hypertension, the most important effect we were trying to achieve, failed to occur.

We felt like throwing in the towel at that point, but instead we tried to identify why the mice's blood pressure did not rise. We returned to test-tube experiments and a few months later realized that human renin did not pair with the mouse counterpart (mouse angiotensinogen). Likewise, mouse renin did not pair with human angiotensinogen. Having confirmed these two points, we mated mice that carried the human renin gene with mice that carried the human angiotensinogen gene. About three months after birth, the offspring of these pairs developed hypertension.

Mice that carried only one of the two factors involved in hypertension did not develop high blood pressure, but when the two were combined in the same mouse, hypertension occurred. Maximum blood pressure in a normal mouse is about 100, but in the hypertensive mice it ranged from 120 to 140. When we administered a renin inhibitor to the hypertensive mice, blood pressure dropped to about 100, and when we stopped administering the medication, blood pressure rose to the previous levels.

Our team then went on to produce "Tsukuba hypotensive mice" by deleting a gene that produces angiotensinogen, closely related to renin. Through this experiment we were attempting to find out if the enzyme/hormone system that triggers renin was really involved in controlling blood pressure at the level of an individual organism. As we had anticipated, the blood pressure of the mice that lacked the gene was thirty points lower than normal mice.

Another Remarkable Discovery

Our research produced a surprising result that surpassed anything I could ever have imagined. One day, the pregnant female mice, which had been mated several times to produce hypertensive mice, developed hypertension. We could understand why their young would have hypertension. After all, they had inherited two hypertensive factors from their parents. But we could not understand why the mother's blood pressure would rise. To determine the cause of this unexpected development, we did a blood test on the females and found human renin, which should have been present only in the male. What did this mean?

At first, we assumed that the hormone must have been transferred during mating. But if that was the case, it should have decomposed within an hour or two. After much investigation, we discovered to our great astonishment that the human renin gene had affected the mother through the placenta. This means that other genes the fetus inherits from the father could also affect the mother during pregnancy. Although we are still at the stage of experimenting on animals, this phenomenon could conceivably occur in humans as well.

In our experiment, the effects ceased as soon as the mother gave birth. As can be seen from figure 10, the blood pressure of the mother at the time of conception (0) increased sharply from the tenth day, peaked just before birth, and returned to normal after birth on the twentieth day. But any functional disorder caused by those genes would have remained. This discovery should help clarify the causes of toxemia in pregnant women.

The results of this experiment were the focus of intense international interest. In November 1996 the prestigious American journal *Science*, which rarely features papers by Japanese scientists, sent a journalist to cover the story and devoted an entire article to our research, hailing our work as the most creative discovery in this field for many years.

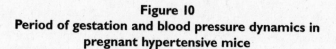

Figure 10
Period of gestation and blood pressure dynamics in pregnant hypertensive mice

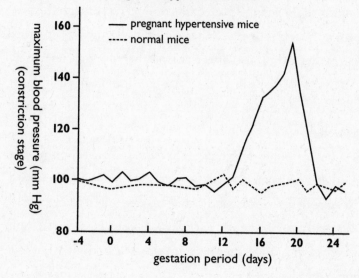

We encountered many setbacks in the years from the planning stage to completion, but studying hypertension in mice was an incredibly rewarding experience. We acquired hypertensive and hypotensive mice, which exhibit two different types of blood pressure, in addition to normal laboratory mice (see figure 11). We are the only research group in the world that has two different types of mice for the study of hypertension. As we do not yet understand the mechanism by

Figure 11
Blood pressure of different mouse types

Type of mouse	Constriction-stage blood pressure (mm Hg)
Tsukuba hypertensive mouse	129.1 ± 7.1
Normal mouse	100.4 ± 4.4
Tsukuba hypotensive mouse	66.9 ± 4.1

Constriction-stage blood pressure is maximum blood pressure.

which hormones raise and lower blood pressure, I believe that the development of these mice will accelerate the study of hypertension. This same technology can be applied to the study and analysis of numerous other diseases, such as cancer.

Although much of the material covered in this chapter may have seemed rather technical, I hope that through it you have gained some insight into the wonders of our genes. The more I study this subject, the more I am amazed by the exquisite system that comprises the human body. The fact that the minuscule information contained in our cells influences our character, behavior, health, and disease has captivated me for my entire career as a scientist, and my awe shows no signs of diminishing. The reality of the blueprint of life is so astounding that I can only assume it to be divine in origin. It makes me keenly aware of the existence of "Something Great," which we will explore in the next chapter.

VI

Uniting Science and the Divine

Advances in Genetic Engineering
Cannot Break Nature's Laws

As science advances, it has become much harder to judge what is useful and what is harmful to society. This is why biotechnology, including genetic engineering, is the focus of so much debate and why the birth of the first cloned sheep in England in 1997 sparked an international controversy. Many people avoid genetically modified foods sold in local supermarkets for fear of health risks, or they question whether human beings have the right to tamper with nature and genes, which are God's creation.

Although genetic modification and cloning both use genetic technology, they are two very different things. But this does not change the fact that genetic engineering directly affects the very mechanism of life. It is therefore impossible to divorce this topic from ethics and religion. The question being asked today is how far should we proceed with genetic-modification technology.

From the perspective of someone involved in genetic research, genetic modification in itself is not bad, as it is something that has always existed. Our ancestors developed improved plant strains because they wanted crops with characteristics favorable for cultivation. The majority of seeds used in agriculture today no longer resemble those of the plants from which they were derived.

The classic method of genetic modification is crossbreeding. Some people are under the false impression that no genetic change takes place through this method. In fact, this conventional method of crop improvement is the epitome of genetic modification, and improved plant hybrids produced through cross-pollination are most definitely genetically modified.

Genetic modification through crossbreeding, however, can only occur between related species. Moreover, harmful genes are transferred along with beneficial genes to the hybrid species and may even dominate. To screen out undesirable genes while retaining desirable ones requires generations of selective breeding, and it is only after many years that a variety with all the desired characteristics can be produced. This same process occurs in the world of nature without any human intervention, which proves that genetic modification per se is not an unnatural act.

More recently, genetic mutation was developed as an alternative to cross-pollination. In this method, plants are bombarded with radiation or toxic chemicals to produce mutations, some of which may have desirable traits. Although this is much faster than cross-pollination, there is no way to control the type of mutation that takes place, and the success rate is very low. Scientists are lucky to obtain one useful mutation out of ten thousand or even several million.

Accordingly, those involved in genetic modification began searching for a quicker, more accurate method. Their efforts bore fruit with the emergence of biotechnology in the 1970s. This technology dramatically reduced the time required to produce new strains and eliminated the need to use related species. It was now possible to genetically modify any kind of seed. At the same time, however, the ability to manipulate genes raised fears that we might produce such monsters as the Chimera, a creature from Greek mythology with the head of a lion, the body of a goat, and the tail of a serpent.

It is true that biotechnology enables us to transfer human genes to mice. It is also technically possible to fuse plant and human cells. But this certainly does not mean that these cells will produce human-plant or human-mouse hybrids. Even if human and plant cells are combined, the genes of one or the other will disappear during the process of cell division. Nature is governed by strict laws. No matter how far biotechnology advances, it will still be impossible to break those fundamental rules.

But why would we seek to transfer genes in the first place? As I explained in chapter 5, genetic transfer can help identify the causes of, and possible cures for, such diseases as cancer or diabetes and allows us to mass-produce substances that are effective in their treatment. Biotechnology has been hailed as a scientific revolution that has applications in a broad range of fields including agriculture, livestock farming, medicine, drug manufacturing, and energy.

Genetic modification does not violate the laws of nature, nor does it make the impossible possible. Rather, it makes possible what was previously highly improbable. A word of caution is necessary, however. Just as healthy foods when eaten in excess can be harmful, this technology has its inherent risks. What it holds for our future will depend on how it is used. At the same time, however, it clearly has tremendous potential to help solve such problems as disease and to contribute to further developments in biology and medicine.

In view of the above, how should we move forward in harmony with nature's laws while doing our best for the good of humanity? In this chapter, I would like to share some of my thoughts on this subject.

Feeling the Presence of Something Great

I am often overcome with a feeling of awe and wonder in my study of genetic information. Who, I wonder, could possibly have written such an exquisite blueprint for life and how did they do it? It seems impossible for information with such complex and extensive meaning to have occurred merely by chance. Therefore, I am forced to acknowledge it as a miracle that far exceeds human understanding or capacity. This leads me to the conclusion that some greater being must exist. For more than a decade I have called this "Something Great."

I once spent several days in the same hotel with Russell L. Schweickart, and we had many opportunities to talk. An American astronaut and a member of the Apollo 9 crew, he shared his experiences in space. I was particularly impressed by one remark he made, the gist of which is this: "The earth from outer space is not just beautiful; it actually seems to be alive. Gazing down at it, I felt myself connected to that life; I felt that I owed my existence to the earth. It was such a moving experience that I cannot express it in words."

Although intellectually we may know that the earth is alive, it is not something we usually register in our daily lives. Schweickart was struck by this realization when looking at the earth from the macrocosmic perspective of outer space. Similarly, I am inspired by the same awe and wonder when I look at the microcosm, the world contained within our genes.

The more I know about genes, the more I am forced to acknowledge their greatness. Our genes, which are contained within the nucleus of cells so small they are invisible, contain three billion combinations of four chemical letters, which are perfectly paired, A with T and C with G. This enormous volume of information is what keeps us alive—and not just us but every living organism on earth from microorganisms to plants, animals, and humans. There are an estimated two million to two hundred million species on this planet, all of which owe their lives to the same genetic code. To me, this seems absolutely incredible, yet it is an indisputable fact. To me, it is truly evidence of the existence of what I call "Something Great."

After his return from outer space, Schweickart was moved to travel the world and share the deep emotion he had experienced with as many people as possible. I, too, am inspired by the same feeling. We cannot define exactly what this "Something Great" is. Some refer to it as the power of Nature; others call it God or Buddha. We are free to define it however we like. But we must never forget that we owe our lives to the workings of this mysterious force.

No matter how determined we are to live, if our genes stop functioning we cannot survive for even one second. The human life span of close to a hundred years is an immeasurable gift from Mother Nature. If someone gave you a million dollars, you would probably be thrilled. You might be a little concerned about taxes, but still you would feel happy. Compared with the gift of life, however, a million dollars is nothing.

We teach our children to be grateful to their parents through whom they are conceived and who nurture them through childhood. I think the majority of people accept the logic in this and are thankful. But as our parents also had parents who again had parents before them, it seems reasonable to me that by extending this gratitude back through previous generations we should eventually reach the parent of all life. Gratitude for our parents should naturally lead to gratitude for those who went before us and therefore to the origin of life. Although we cannot see it, the continuity of life indicates that such an entity exists. Working in genetic research has gradually made me realize how important it is to fix our gaze firmly on the fact that we owe our lives to this existence, which transcends our own.

Do Genes Have a Soul?

My life's work as a genetic scientist has led me to certain beliefs regarding what happens to us after we die. Life has continuity. A parent's genes are transmitted to the child and the child's to the grandchild, and so life continues. However, it is only the continuity of genes, not of life, that can be confirmed. Genes are not synonymous with life. They are only the blueprint, the design rather than the reality. If life is not found in our genes, then where and what is it? We do not know. Once we have read the meaning of the decoded human genome, I am sure that we will understand more, but I expect that we will still be unable to precisely define the essence of life.

Many believe that when we die we are reincarnated. They believe that the individual has a soul, which is manifest in the physical world when it resides in the body. Reincarnation refers to the continuity of this soul. Although the soul cannot be defined, according to this concept, it is eternal, and therefore when the flesh perishes, the soul leaves the body and reappears within another.

I do not know whether or not this is true, but I do know that such things cannot be explained at the genetic level. Genes are material, and it is impossible to describe the soul in material terms. Just because we cannot explain it, however, does not mean that it does not exist. As I see it, the soul is not something of which I can be consciously aware. Generally, that of which I am conscious is "mind," not soul. The mind feels happiness, sadness, and anger, but when the body dies, it cannot continue to exist. As the mind belongs to the conscious world, it is inseparable from the flesh and therefore must perish with the body. The unconscious world, on the other hand, is beyond human awareness. The soul is connected to this realm and, through it, to the world of Something Great. Therefore, although my soul exists, I am usually not consciously aware of it. This is why the world of the divine has always been impossible to understand within the context of reason and consciousness alone.

In his book *The Astonishing Hypothesis: The Scientific Search for the Soul* (New York: Charles Scribner's Sons, 1994), Francis Crick, who along with James Watson proposed the helical structure for DNA, concludes that genes do not have a soul. Genes transmit the physical continuity of human beings, but the soul appears to belong to a different dimension. Even if we decode every gene, we still will not understand the soul. It is a subject that, perhaps fittingly, will always be a divine mystery to us.

One factor that hinders our quest for understanding is the tendency to confuse the concepts of mind and soul. Clearly distinguishing between the two—that the mind is of the body and the soul is of Something Great—makes it easier to understand the issue of life and death. The soul, as the source of our existence, is essential, but as long as we live in the physical world, so too are the mind and the body, without which we could not exist in this world. The understanding that both the mind and the soul are intimately related to the genetic blueprint of life can help us discover the best way of interacting with our genes to live up to our potential.

We Are Far More Wonderful Than We Think

The composition of our body is exquisite. Each person has far more ability than they could ever imagine, but the fact that few people realize this is not so strange. Although modern scientific developments have given us intellectual understanding of the body's amazing structure, it is still difficult for us to register the true significance of this in our daily lives. It hit Schweickart for the first time when he was gazing down at the earth from outer space. I, too, am only beginning to catch a glimmer through my work with genes. But as most of us never have the opportunity to encounter the microcosmic or macrocosmic reality, it is only natural that it is difficult to really grasp what it means. Not everyone can travel in space, nor can I show you your genes. Instead, let me share another story that proves we are far more wonderful than we imagine.

Have you ever heard of a single tomato plant producing twelve thousand tomatoes? Such plants were exhibited at the Tsukuba Science and Technology Expo in 1985. Most people assumed that they were the product of biotechnology, but in fact they were produced from the seeds of an ordinary tomato variety that normally would produce only twenty or thirty tomatoes. If not biotechnology, then what was their secret? The plants were cultivated by the hydroponic method using sunlight and nutrient-enriched water. The only difference was that they were grown in water rather than in soil.

Normally, soil is essential for plant cultivation. Plants send their roots into the ground to absorb the nutrients and moisture they need to grow. Of course, they need sunlight and air as well, but soil has always been regarded as one of the most important aspects of cultivation. Agronomist Shigeo Nozawa, however, thought that the opposite was true. Believing that a plant's inherent capacity for growth is inhibited by the fact that its roots grow in soil, he grew the plants in water, releasing the roots from their confinement and allowing them to freely absorb nature's gifts. This is known as the hydroponic method, and the result was tomato plants that bore a thousand times more fruit than conventional plants. Nozawa was able to view life from the perspective of a tomato plant. From this, we can see that even tomatoes have potential far beyond what we imagine. If Nozawa's philosophy helped plants realize their potential, what would happen if we applied this philosophy to human beings?

Although we strive to develop our potential, we remain trapped within our perception of limitations. If our parents or teachers say, "Couldn't you get better grades than that?" we are likely to answer, "That was the best I could do." These perceived limitations are almost always based on comparison with other people, which is an extremely limited point of view. Still, we are convinced that they exist, and we see our own experience and knowledge as absolute. This is a very narrow perspective.

Nozawa explained how he got the idea for producing giant tomatoes: "The plants we see around us are expressing only limited potential in response to certain conditions. I began to examine what conditions were preventing them from realizing greater potential. I came to the conclusion that soil was one of the obstacles." According to conventional wisdom, soil is necessary for plant growth, but Nozawa turned this idea upside down. Plants may send out roots, but soil gets in their way. Water changes frequently when in natural soil. In addition, soil obstructs the supply of enzymes and directly exposes plants to changes in temperature. Physiological changes are the result of chemical reactions, and obstacles such as soil interfere with this process. Nozawa concluded that if these restrictions were removed, the efficiency of photosynthesis would be improved and plant growth would be accelerated. His theory was verified by a thousandfold increase in yield in his tomato plants.

Human beings are the same. If we remove all obstacles and provide an appropriate environment, our potential for development is limitless. If tomatoes can achieve a thousandfold increase in potential, then it would not be unrealistic to expect an even greater increase in the abilities of human beings, which are more complex organisms. I took my students to stand by Nozawa's giant tomato plants. "If tomatoes can do this," I told them, "then you have even greater potential."

Nozawa claimed that soil inhibits plant growth. What are the factors inhibiting the development of human potential? One that might spring to mind for many people is self-gratification. Everyone knows that drinking, gambling, and sexual immorality are not good for us. But the issue is not so simple. A moderate amount of some alcoholic beverages can be beneficial to health, and gambling in some cases can help relieve stress. If the pleasure we seek is sex, it is infidelity, promiscuity, and prostitution that are harmful, not sexual desire itself.

Rather than self-gratification, the main factor inhibiting human potential is our way of thinking. What type of thinking is harmful? Negative thinking that violates the laws of nature. As people have many different value systems, there is not necessarily a single uniform standard of right and wrong. Some people will see a certain act or event as good while others will see it as bad. This discrepancy occurs frequently in daily life. Therefore, the definition of the "right way to live" will differ from one person to the next, and to debate the subject will only lead to further confusion.

One immutable fact remains: our genes and the way they function. When they are in harmony with the laws of nature, they work to protect and nurture life and rejoice in it. Therefore, I think that we need to look more closely at nature and strive to live in harmony with its laws. If we can do this, then

I think that—like the tomato plants—we will be able to tap the incredible potential within us.

Live in Harmony

It is easy to say that we should live in harmony with the laws of nature, but we do not know all of those laws. Moreover, our perceptions of what living in harmony means may very well be biased, and they will certainly differ from one person to the next. In the past, religion taught us how we should live, but today many are alienated by religion and have placed their faith in science instead.

Science has made remarkable advances over the last century, and medicine appears to have conquered many diseases, yet we still cannot cure cancer or clearly identify the cause of hypertension. In the case of hypertension, we have made definite advances in this field. However, although we can lower blood pressure, we still cannot cure hypertension because we only understand a very small part of the mechanism that causes it. The full picture remains shrouded in mystery. Likewise, the mechanisms causing the majority of lifestyle diseases have not yet been identified. Thus, we cannot claim that modern medicine is effectively curing disease.

People are free to put their faith in science if they choose, but I do not think that science alone can solve everything. At the same time, the rift between religion and science continues to widen, and modern people accustomed to scientific thought are no longer convinced by religious precepts. Personally, I see both science and religion as originating from the same source, and therefore I seek some way to reconcile them. It is no longer possible in this modern age to accept a religion encumbered by the traditions of a bygone era, but at the same time, we cannot place complete faith in science.

So what can we do? I have three suggestions that I have found helpful in my own life. They are (1) to have noble intentions, (2) to live with an attitude of thankfulness, and (3) to think positively.

Keep Your Intentions Noble

The first proposal, to have noble intentions, is one that has had a profound impact on my life. As I have already related, several times in my study of renin I was fortunate to be the first to achieve certain results. But the subjects that my research team and I chose initially appeared impossible. Why would I become involved in studying subjects that common sense dictated were better avoided? In the beginning, I was driven by my pride as a scientist, ambition, and the desire to improve myself, but this gradually changed as I began to examine genes more closely and became aware of the existence of Something Great. Yes, it was a thrill to compete with the world's top scientists, but my choices were also based on my growing conviction that striving toward noble intentions would please Something Great.

As I have said before, this is not an entity I can rationally understand. But when I trace the long continuum of life passed down through our genes from previous generations, it leads me to the conclusion that there must be an original parent. Surely, even if I am not the brightest of children, this parent will be pleased with my efforts to be of service to others, however small my contribution may be. When I began to act on this belief, events began occurring in my life which convinced me that my intentions were acknowledged. The results of our efforts began to bear fruit in a way which made me feel that Something Great was watching over us. Through my experiences in studying genes I came to realize that if we can learn to live with our good genes switched on, we can tap potential far beyond the ordinary.

Live with an Attitude of Thankfulness

My second proposal is to live with an attitude of thankfulness. Life is full of ups and downs. Sometimes it seems impossible to have noble intentions. What can we do to keep ourselves enthusiastic at such times? For me, it helps to remember that we do not live by our own strength and ingenuity alone but rather through the priceless gift conferred on us by nature. We can be thankful just for the fact that we are alive each day.

My study of genes has shown me that our existence itself is a marvelous wonder. This is particularly clear when I observe the relationship between the individual cell and the organism as a whole. We are comprised of sixty trillion cells, which through a highly sophisticated order make up the organs, tissues, and other parts of the body. Just look at a liver cell, for example. Only those genes necessary for it to function as an individual cell are switched on, yet at the same time, it forms part of the liver. This is like an employee working in a company. The employee carries out a specific job for that company but at the same time is not subordinate. The employee has an individual life of his or her own. A cell is the same. On the one hand, it may function as a liver cell, but on the other, it has its own individuality and functions within the organ autonomously and selectively.

Let's examine this relationship from the perspective of the kidney. The kidney plays an important role in regulating liquids and salt. In an adult, it circulates one hundred and fifty liters of blood per day from the main artery. As the blood vessels approach the center of the kidney, they become thinner. A blood-filtering mechanism located at the tip of each blood vessel filters out waste such as urine and absorbs necessary elements. The enzyme renin, which I have been studying, is found in certain kidney cells. Thus, although the kidney is an independent organ, it is comprised of individual cells with different functions, including blood vessels of various sizes and filtering mechanisms, and these combine to form the kidney, working together to perform a vital function within the human body. If we look at the individual cells comprising it, we find that while they faithfully carry out their duties for the kidney, each cell also efficiently and independently performs such functions as cell maintenance and repair, which are related solely to the individual cell. If each cell in a blood vessel did not work autonomously, for example, the blood vessel's lattice-like pattern could not be constantly repaired. Yet when cells combine to form a blood vessel, they regulate their speed of cell division and their shape with that of other cells. While the cell forms just one part, it is furnished with the characteristics of the whole. This is true not only for the relationship between cells and the kidney but also for that between people and society, people and the earth, or people and the universe. We are all a part of the universe. We live within the order of nature on this planet, yet at the same time, we are participating in the creation of that order. We are participating fully just by living.

The Darwinian theory of evolution has dominated modern society. According to this theory, we evolved through natural selection and mutation and only the fittest survived. Survival of the fittest was assumed to be a law of nature, a law whereby only the victors could enjoy life. Life was viewed as a constant competition, and where there is competition there will always be some who win and some who lose. This means that roughly half the human race will be winners and the remaining half will inevitably be losers who should be screened out.

In the 1960s, however, Boston University biologist Lynn Margulis proposed a different theory of evolution. Known as the Endosymbiotic Theory, it is based on the idea that life evolved through mutual cooperation rather than through survival of the fittest. This theory explains the process of evolution in detail beginning with the first living creatures, which were single-cell organisms without a nucleus such as in the E. coli bacteria. The union of several simple cells or cell parts that worked together to make a new type of cell achieved evolution to the next level—cells with a nucleus.

Although this theory focuses on the cellular level, there is an interesting parallel at the human level. In the prevailing Darwinian view, humanity passed through various stages in evolution from apes to primitive man by following the "law of the jungle." However, according to an archaeologist who studied 150-million-year-old remains of anthropoid apes found at Lake Turkana in Kenya, there is evidence that the apes shared food and helped each other but no evidence of the strong oppressing the weak or of conflicts among them. If we are to believe Darwinian theory, we evolved through a process of conflict. Yet more recent theories suggest that symbiotic cooperation may have been more like it. Research about the way in which genes function also indicates that the latter theories are more compatible with the laws of nature.

When I look at life in this way, it seems only natural to thank Something Great for the bounty of being alive. Each human being, just by being born, becomes a participant in life. Regardless of the results, there is value just in being here. I personally think that this is something to be thankful for. Although some people may disagree, this attitude can make life much more fun. To live with gratitude is to be thankful to be alive. Living with an attitude of thankfulness allows us to appreciate and enjoy each day, regardless of whether or not anything special happens.

Keep Your Thoughts Positive

My third suggestion—which I believe is the most important—is to think positively. Life does not always unfold according to our wishes. We get sick, make mistakes, or suffer a broken heart. In my case, I frequently face setbacks such as being beaten at research, and I am often confronted with situations that seem impossible. But no matter how bad a situation appears, it is important to see it in a positive rather than a negative light. In fact, it is during times of hardship when everything seems to go wrong that we particularly need a positive attitude. This means developing the ability to discern meaning even in the most terrible hardship, to see the things that happen to us as a message or a gift. If you think this is impossible, just remember that Something Great, the parent of all parents, would never harm us—because we are its children. This does not mean that we never experience tragedies but rather that we should look for the lesson or goodness which comes from unfortunate events. This perspective can help us to accept whatever comes our way and to see crisis as an opportunity. I make this suggestion on the basis of fact. As I have explained, positive thinking can turn on our genes, stimulating our brain and body to produce beneficial hormones. From my own experience, I feel certain that this is true.

There are two sides to everything: front and back, night and day, strength and weakness. No matter how one-sided something appears, no matter how final it looks, there is always room for choice. Take the disease AIDS, for example. Some people take the fatalistic view that AIDS is divine punishment for sexual immorality. Looked at in the broader sense, there are very few periods in human history in which sexual immorality was absent, and when it was, people were usually suffering from much worse disasters or misfortunes such as famine, war, or plague. These were dark times in which culture stagnated and people were under a dark cloud. If sexual immorality is not a product of the modern age, then I think it is somewhat illogical to blame AIDS on this alone. Instead, I propose a different perspective.

AIDS is completely different from any other disease we have known. The AIDS virus does not directly kill the person who has it; rather, it destroys the body's natural defense mechanism. Because it attacks and destroys the stronghold of the immune system, the patient contracts and dies from diseases that others would not catch or that are not normally fatal.

The human body comes equipped with an impressive defense system. The world is full of bacteria, and although we cannot see them, we are constantly bombarded by disease-carrying germs. They enter our body in droves. If any survive once inside and multiply until they reach a certain number, we get sick. Usually, however, our immune system kicks in to destroy them before this can happen. This system has an amazing arsenal of antibodies that can destroy millions of germs entering the body at one time.

Antibodies usually fight germs one on one, which means that our bodies have enough antibodies to individually attack and destroy every one of the germs. Of course, this could not be done without our genes. Every gene has the instructions for combating millions of germs. But how do they know how to respond when there is no telling what kind of germ will enter the body? Do they already have all the information for every type of germ? This question puzzled scientists in the field of immunology for many years. The Japanese Nobel Prize laureate Susumu Tonegawa, who works in the United States, made a major contribution to solving it. The mechanism functions like this: genetic information is divided into parts that can be combined in any way necessary to make antibodies which respond to specific germs. Although there are a limited variety of components, millions of antibodies can be made through different combinations to protect the body against invasion by most types of germs.

It was through the emergence of AIDS that we learned what a marvelous system protects us from disease. Even in the face of an illness like this, we should not despair. Rather, we should take the positive attitude that it can be cured. In fact, many cases exist in which a patient's mental attitude during treatment affected the onset of AIDS. Although positive thinking may seem difficult, negative thinking could very well be detrimental to your genes. A positive attitude is the most important factor in influencing our genes, no matter how negative the situation.

Genes Are Both Bold and Tenacious

Just as I said, everything has two sides, and genes also have two sides that enable them to fulfill two important yet contradictory jobs. One job is to transmit genetic information accurately from parent to child. To do this, genetic information must remain stable. Like the family precepts that successfully carry a family business through several generations, the genetic information transmitted to our descendants must be constant. The other job is the daily maintenance of the cell as an individual organism. The external world surrounding it, however, is always in a state of flux. It is impossible to adapt to changes in the natural world if the organism remains absolutely immutable. Thus, there are times when genetic recombination may be necessary.

Genes fulfill these two conflicting roles beautifully by forming a double-helix structure. To put it simply, this structure results in a substantial amount of "wasted" space inside the DNA, making it possible for our genes to easily maintain an unchanging stability and at the same time to make drastic changes should the need arise. Our genes can deftly use the on/off mechanism to respond as needed to external stimuli.

Genes teach us a valuable lesson from this characteristic: the need to be both bold and tenacious. Being bold means being able to break through conventional methods and customs when necessary. In my case, I had to make bold decisions countless times during my study of renin. For example, when deciphering the genetic code, I took the drastic step of introducing genetic engineering, which was just emerging, because it was clear that we could not possibly succeed using conventional methods. This technology had almost never been used in this field, but because I dared to try it, we were the first to decode human renin. If I had vacillated because there was no precedent or because I was an amateur in the field, I and the other members of the group would have lost a precious opportunity to develop as scientists. Taking bold steps like these resembles what happens at the cellular level when genes radically recombine in response to changes in the environment.

As for tenacity, I do not mean clinging to conventional methods and being resistant to change but rather following through on your heart's desire. In my case, for example, I have a tenacious attachment to the study of renin. I have not changed the topic of my research for over twenty years. But I have changed the level at which I studied it, beginning with molecules and then progressing to the cell and from the cell to the organism. This tenacity enabled me to boldly introduce the latest technology from genetic engineering to embryo-logical engineering. I have also stuck tenaciously to my original conviction that our research must succeed because of the useful contributions it will make.

Genes likewise are tenacious in their commitment to transmitting genetic information to subsequent generations. This is what drives them to work so hard to maintain the cell and to proliferate, even to the extent of a gene sacrificing itself to survive as a whole. In other words, tenacity can actually generate flexibility and the willingness to drastically change methods in order to achieve an objective.

People have a tendency to think that when there are two options, they must choose one over the other. But genes, the blueprint of all life, are not made this way. Some sections of a gene known as *exons* are encoded with specific instructions while other sections known as *introns* do not encode any instructions and appear to be wasted space. Yet genetic information contains far more introns than exons. Thus, rather than selecting one option and rejecting another, nature chooses symbiotic coexistence. In the same way, boldness and tenacity are both necessary. We have much to learn from this characteristic of our genes that is relevant to both society and our way of life.

Everything That Happens to Us Is Necessary

We often talk about good luck and bad and worry about whether luck is on our side. We also frequently speak of coincidence or chance. We use these expressions to describe the incomprehensible—things that we cannot control. I believe, however, that everything which happens to us is necessary, both the good and the bad, and this belief is based on experiences that date back to my childhood.

When I was growing up, Japan was very poor and my family was particularly poor. My parents could not buy me toys, and when I was in high school they could not afford to send me on a particular school trip. My grandfather had died many years earlier, and my grandmother, who lived with us, was the head of the family. She had a habit of saying, "Our savings are in heaven." My mother said the same thing: "I know you feel bad about the school trip, but don't worry. We've deposited that trip in heaven's account. In the future, I'm sure you'll be able to travel all over the world." They assured me that whatever I did to help others would be returned a thousandfold and that it did not matter whether it happened in my own lifetime or in that of my children or grandchildren, because my life was connected to those of successive generations. As I was still a child, this explanation failed to satisfy me, and I often wished that they would set aside some savings for me here and now, not just in heaven. In retrospect, however, I can see that my mother's words came true. I traveled to America to study when it was still very difficult for Japanese to go abroad, and I have been overseas many times since that time.

By "depositing our savings in heaven," they meant that money should be used not just for oneself but also for the betterment of the world. We do not always get to see the results of our actions. Doing good deeds often requires sacrifice. It is the part we sacrifice that we have deposited in heaven's bank, and it is returned in the future to you or to others as a natural outcome. It is like planting a tree that will not bear fruit until you are dead, but you do it because you know that other generations will enjoy it, and the joy in that knowledge is your reward along with the fruits of trees planted by your ancestors which you are now enjoying. Or think of a farmer sowing seeds. Farmers prepare the land for the spring sowing before winter by spreading plenty of manure and tilling the earth. If you want a bountiful harvest, you have to prepare for it, and if you fail to do so, you will not have any yield the next year. Life is the same. No matter how difficult, it is necessary to prepare the ground before sowing your seeds.

Why did my grandmother do this? I think she was inspired by an awareness of Something Great and the belief that if you continuously strive to do the right thing, you will be blessed. Although some people may doubt this, I do not, because I have experienced the truth of it myself. No goal can be achieved without spending time and sometimes seemingly unrequited effort in preparation. If we become discouraged during this process, it is because we lack conviction. Conversely, if we have unswerving faith in the outcome, we will never give up. To persevere is the greatest secret of success. It is not easy, however, to have confidence. We may think we have it only to find it shaken later. To prevent this, we must fix our sights not on the immediate future but on the larger perspective, believing that nothing is impossible. To have unshakable faith, we need to take pride in what we have achieved so far.

Maintaining the Balance of Nature's Laws

In a previous section, I introduced the high-yield hyponica tomato plant as evidence of the tremendous potential latent within plants and, likewise, humans. Yet this example brings up another question: Why doesn't this phenomenon occur in tomatoes that grow naturally? Personally, I think that it is due to the principle of "self-restraint."

For each specific environment, nature has determined an appropriate number. If one species of animal exceeds a certain number, the population will always begin to decline. All living creatures maintain the appropriate number for survival in that environment.

This phenomenon is also found in genes. According to some scientists, certain genes are egotistic, pursuing only their own profit, which for a gene is survival and proliferation, while others are altruistic, urging cells toward self-sacrifice and death. What causes this seeming contradiction between survival and death? Once again, it is the principle of self-restraint. If genes continued to proliferate and never died, it would result in a disastrous explosion in numbers. Living organisms must eat to survive, but if there are too many, there will not be enough food. Nor will there be enough space to accommodate them all. Therefore, our genes are programmed to maintain an appropriate scale, and death is an essential part of this process. As living things must die, we need both egotistic and altruistic genes. This is the mechanism that maintains balance for the entire planet.

In contrast, a look at human behavior suggests that we lost the art of self-restraint as history advanced toward the modern age. We have depleted oil and gas reserves to the point of exhaustion, stripped lands of their forests without any regard for their ecosystems, and applied toxic agrochemicals in pursuit of ever-greater yields. Such actions, which can only be described as human arrogance, are becoming increasingly conspicuous. As I pointed out earlier, we need unshakable confidence, but if we are not careful, this can lead to arrogance. When that danger rears its head, I suggest that we should recall the altruistic side of our genetic makeup and practice self-restraint, an attitude in agreement with the laws of nature.

Perhaps tomato plants in nature do not bear twelve thousand tomatoes because there is no need or because there is some reason that they should not. Biotechnology has tremendous potential, but if we are to use that technology effectively, self-restraint is essential. This is true not only for biotechnology but for all branches of science. It is important to refrain from violating the laws of nature by destruction of the natural environment or by altering the form of living creatures, even if technology makes it possible.

After laying its eggs, a certain type of moth with protective coloring flies about until it exhausts all its energy and dies. To us this seems like suicide, but by doing so, it robs predators of the opportunity to learn how to spot other moths of the same species. Another type of moth that is poisonous remains motionless after laying its eggs, making it easy prey for predators. It is believed that by doing so, they teach predators that they are not tasty and in that way they protect their young. Although these adult moths could live longer if they chose, they sacrifice their lives for the future of their species. They consider no other alternative.

We humans could learn much from this obedience to the laws of nature. If we do not, we will jeopardize the future of the human race, for we can never hope to transcend nature's laws, no matter how hard we may try.

In the past, I found it hard to grasp what people meant when they talked about a being or force that transcends humankind. Some call it God and others call it Buddha. But while studying genes, which are only one part of its creation, I sensed its existence and was profoundly moved. True self-restraint is born from the knowledge of the existence of Something Great, and awareness of it can help us grow tremendously as human beings.

There are many things that we still do not understand about life. My dream is to continue exploring the essence of life not only from the scientific point of view but also from a spiritual and religious perspective.